Surviving the Cold and Flu Season Naturally

Faith A. Christensen, ND

Colorado Natural Health, Inc.
Colorado Springs, Colorado

Published by:

Colorado Natural Health, Inc.

620 South Cascade Ste 110

Colorado Springs, CO 80906

719-685-2500

Printed in the United States of America

5 4 3 2 1

Acknowledgments

I am especially grateful to:

My family for all the support they have given me, especially while writing this book. My sisters who generously volunteered childcare services in order to write this book. In particular, I want to thank my parents for the inspiration and encouragement to publish this book and my father, Neal, for his editing expertise. Christine Riggin, ND for her insightful additions and support. Jean Christensen for her wonderful editing and organizational efforts. Casey Wait for her beautiful mullein drawing for the cover image. Anne Elizabeth South for editing the second edition. Bastyr University for the excellent education and drive to combine science with nature that leads to science based natural medicine.

Table of Contents

1 | Why Survive Naturally?

Most of us dread the onset of the "cold and flu" season especially if we have young children or are prone to catch just about any "bug" wafting our way. Since most colds and all flus are viral in nature, modern medicine does not have a "pill" to cure the common cold or flu. The best modern medicine can offer is vaccinations and anti-viral medications with substantial side effects. Over the counter "cold and flu" medicine only address symptoms and not root causes of an illness and most suppress the body's natural defense against these invaders.

In addition, antibiotics prescribed incorrectly for viral infections cause an increase in antibiotic-resistant strains of bacteria. The Center for Disease Control estimates more than 10 million courses of antibiotics are prescribed each year for viral conditions which never benefit from antibiotics, because antibiotics address bacteria and not viruses.[1]

Ear infections, pharyngitis, bronchitis, and the common cold are often treated with antibiotics when the majority of these cases are not bacterial but viral. According to the Center for Disease Control, children and healthy adults under 50 years old receive most of the inappropriate antibiotic prescriptions.

Adverse Antibiotic Effects

Antibiotic resistant bacteria: When bacteria are faced with antibiotics, they attempt to survive by mutating to outsmart the antibiotic's killing mechanism. The resulting trend is the number of antibiotic-resistant bacteria continues to rise yearly. The Institute of Medicine has identified antibiotic resistance as one of the key microbial threats to health in the United States. [2]

Destruction of friendly bacteria: Since antibiotics do not distinguish which bacteria they kill, they often destroy friendly bacteria as well as the invading bacteria. Friendly bacteria are an important component of a healthy body. They help convert hormones, protect against inflammation, and support immune function in the digestive tract. For example, regulation of estrogen is dependent on friendly bacteria converting inactive estrogen secreted by the gall bladder into active estrogen to maintain proper levels. When friendly bacteria are destroyed by antibiotics this recycling of estrogen does not occur making some birth control pills ineffective.

Yeast overgrowth: Antibiotics can cause an overgrowth of yeast by killing friendly bacteria in the digestive tract. With the removal of friendly bacteria, there is more room in the digestive tract and available food for yeast to thrive on. Overgrowth of yeast causes immune suppression and a greater risk of developing future infections. An overgrowth of yeast can also increase inflammation in the digestive tract and lead to the development of food allergies.

Immune suppression: Treatment with antibiotics often increases the likelihood of repeat infections, especially with repeated use, because of the destruction of friendly bacteria and decreased memory cell and immunoglobulin production due to a shortened immune response. When an antibiotic is introduced at the onset of an infection, its killing activity works quickly and decreases the immune system's opportunity to mount a full attack.

Nutrient loss: Because a course of antibiotics can cause digestive irritation, diarrhea or dysfunctional intestinal flora, vital nutrients needed to support the immune system function are lost.

Allergic reactions: Allergic reactions are often associated with antibiotic use. Most of the time the reaction involves skin rashes and swelling, but some reactions are more deadly.

With the significant increase in antibiotic resistant infections as well as the negative effects of antibiotic use, surviving the cold and flu season without taking an antibiotic is a win-win situation for everyone. In addition, immune-strengthening lifestyle and nutrition habits improve your overall health and can help prevent serious health conditions such as Type II diabetes, cancer, and heart disease.

To Survive the Cold and Flu Season Naturally
- Decrease exposure to bacteria and viruses
- Decrease immune-suppressive activities
- Increase dietary and lifestyle habits to support and boost the immune system
- Take immune-supportive herbs before and after an illness for prevention and recovery
- Take appropriate herbs, homeopathics, vitamins/minerals to boost the immune system when exposed
- Allow the immune system to do its job when sick and give it specific support

You can survive the cold and flu season naturally. Your body has tremendous infection fighting capability. All it needs is a little help from you!

---

[1] National Center for Immunization and Respiratory Diseases/Division of Bacterial Diseases. (2006). *Get smart: Know when antibiotics work.* Retrieved January 23, 2007, from http://www.cdc.gov/drugresistance/community/anitbiotic-resistance.htm.

[2] National Center for Immunization and Respiratory Diseases/Division of Bacterial Diseases. (2006). *Get smart: Know when antibiotics work.* Retrieved January 23, 2007, from http://www.cdc.gov/drugresistance/community/anitbiotic-resistance.htm.

2 | Meet the Natural Defense Team- Your Immune System

The immune system is a powerful "army" comprised of fighter cells, killer cells, chemical messengers, and chemical fighters. This intricate system also communicates with the nervous system and endocrine (hormone) system of the body creating a complex and highly refined network.

White Blood Cells

White blood cells are the hard-working soldiers on the front lines. These cells patrol the bloodstream and entryways of the body (eyes, ears, nose, mouth, ears, etc.), to help prevent germs from invading the body. Since white blood cells are able to squeeze through tiny blood vessels, they can leave the bloodstream to enter other tissues being attacked by foreign invaders.

There are millions of white blood cells in each drop of blood. There are also many specialized units called lymphocytes, macrophages, monocytes, eosinophils, and basophils. If the main white blood cell troops become overwhelmed, the specialists jump into action to provide more specific support.

If viruses enter the body and begin to multiply, lymphocytes step in to more effectively eliminate the viruses. Lymphocytes gather key information about the invading virus and return to the lymph glands to teach other lymphocytes how to kill the specific virus. When this team is activated, lymph nodes and tonsils become enlarged and painful due to increased activity of lymphocyte training, recruitment, and killing action.

The main control station for lymphocytes is the thymus, a tiny gland in front of the heart. Lymphocytes train and mature in the thymus before going out to all the lymph nodes.

If lymphocytes are overrun by an infection, a special SWAT team called killer lymphocytes or natural killer cells comes to the rescue. Natural killer cells play an important role in searching out pre-cancerous cells, bacteria, and viruses everywhere in the body to protect against full-blown infection and developing cancer.

If bacteria overrun the lymphocyte first line of defense, macrophages (meaning big eater) search out every place in the body to gobble up harmful invaders. They contain huge amounts of chemicals that empower them to digest anything they eat.

Basophils and Eosinophils (specialized groups of white blood cells) spring into action when you have allergies or a parasite infection. They release many different chemicals that start the cascade of an inflammatory reaction.

Chemical messengers and fighters

The immune system has a magnificent communication system. If any invader is detected either through the skin or an infection in the throat, white blood cells send out chemical messengers to mobilize the rest of the team and direct them to the area of infection.

Once the white blood cells reach the battle, they produce chemical fighters, known as cytokines. Cytokines dilate the blood vessels, causing more blood flow and enabling more white blood cells to enter the infected area.

One powerful cytokine, interferon, signals command headquarters to tell the brain the body needs to rest. This conserves energy to allow the body to concentrate on the battle against the disease. Cytokine messengers also tell the body to hold onto immune boosting nutrients such as zinc and vitamin C.

Chemical Weapons

White blood cells have a number of chemical weapons available. They can shoot gamma-interferon into invaders like a poisonous arrow that interferes with the germ's ability to reproduce itself. Specialized white blood cells called B-cells produce antibodies that seek out and attach to specific germs. Some of these antibodies, called immunoglobulins, poke holes in the germs and cause their death

Other antibodies act like chemical glue, making the germs stick together so they can be rounded up and eliminated by white blood cells. Some antibodies, such as secretory IgA, line the mucous passages of the mouth, throat and digestive tract. Secretory IgA attaches to bacteria and allergens and prevents their invasion into the tissues.

Immune Memory

The immune system is remarkable in its ability to remember every past battle and learn from experience. If the same (or similar) germ attacks again, the white blood cells are ready for it. Your body recognizes the invader and remembers how to attack it, ensuring victory every time if the immune system is properly supported.

Because the immune system has an extensive memory, getting sick every once in a while trains the immune system to perform even better. This is especially true for children. A young immune system develops from exposure to germs and training during infections. Most of the immune training actually occurs in the digestive tract since fifty percent of the immune system is located within this system. It is here that the immune system learns the difference between food and invaders. It creates many memory cells against common bacteria, viruses, and parasites found in food and drinking water.

Hygiene Hypothesis

Certain asthma and allergic conditions are now thought to be partially due to overly strict hygiene conditions which deprive the immune system of training missions and create an immune system that is hyper-responsive to dust, pollen and other inert particles. Exposure to microbes may initiate protective responses and play a critical role in the shaping of the immune response when encountered at important early stages during the maturation of immune responses. This could result in the development of immune tolerance to potential allergens. A major basis for the hypothesis is that improved hygienic conditions in developed countries results in less microbial exposure during early but critical time periods in early childhood.[1]

For example, the introduction of bleach has significantly reduced the number of viruses and bacteria that children come into contact with. This creates a lack of training for the immune system and may result in an immune system that reacts to everything even if it is not a threat.

Immunization

The concept of immune memory is the rationale behind immunizations. A small dose of a dead or weakened virus given in an immunization sets up a training exercise for the immune system. Your body uses the lessons learned during training to overcome threats from live viruses.

Most of the time, actually getting a disease provides lifelong immunity, whereas immunizations require boosters to provide a longer immunity. For diseases such as chickenpox which have a very low mortality rate, getting the virus itself provides more protection than the vaccination.

Vaccinations are required every few months for infants because their immune system is still developing and does not hold onto the memory of the vaccine for very long.

One immunological concern with vaccinations is that many different virus particles are given at the same time. Often an infant will have over 6 virus or bacterial particles given to them in one visit. This would be overwhelming to anyone's system, let alone an infant with an underdeveloped immune system.

Smart Viruses

The herpes virus and HIV are particularly adept at evading attacks from the immune system. The herpes virus hides out in tissues for long periods of time, and only comes out when immune system defenses are down. Then it retreats back into its hideout, lying dormant for months or years before it wages another attack. Some viruses, such as HIV, hide within the immune system itself, infiltrating the ranks and destroying the immune system from within.

When Things Go Wrong

Sometimes the immune system attacks the very organs it is supposed to defend. These conditions are called auto-immune diseases because the immune system attacks itself. Examples of this are rheumatoid arthritis (antibodies attacking tissues of the joints), diabetes (antibodies attacking insulin-producing cells in the pancreas), and multiple sclerosis (in which the immune system may be attacking the myelin sheath of the nerves).

There are times when the immune system overreacts, causing a hypersensitive response. This hypersensitive response is often triggered by an allergy. The white blood cells engulf the invading allergen, such as a particle of pollen in the air and release too many chemicals which cause other problems, such as wheezing, rashes, or swelling.

The fact that the immune system views pollen, dust, food or animal dander as an invader is in itself a malfunction. It's an indication the immune system is overly active and tends to view more ordinary things as invaders rather than being on the alert only for true threats to the system.

For all of these situations, retraining the immune system through immuno-modulating herbs and supporting it through proper immune supportive nutrition can effectively change the disease process.

Hormones and the Immune System

Numerous interactions exist among the nervous, endocrine and immune systems, mediated by neurotransmitters, hormones and cytokines. Each system of the body produces chemical messengers to communicate with the other systems and regulate its function.[2] For example, immune cells can produce thyroid stimulating hormone that directly interacts with thyroid hormone production.[3]

The hormones secreted or regulated by the pituitary gland regulate every level of immune activity. These main hormones of the body are secreted in pulses related to sleep wake cycles and the age-related decline of immune function.[4] Prolactin, growth hormone and thyroid hormones act to protect against stress-induced suppression in immune function by boosting immune activity during times of stress. Furthermore, hormone deficiencies correlate with a decline in immune function and other systems.[5] Consequently, identifying and treating hormonal deficiencies is an important part of supporting ideal immune system functioning.

DHEA

DHEA (dehydroepiandrosterone) is the most plentiful hormone in the body and can be converted to estrogen and testosterone. DHEA usually starts to decline after age thirty, with large amounts of stress accelerating the natural decline of DHEA. DHEA supplementation of 50 mg for 20 weeks in elderly men with deficient DHEA demonstrated an increase in monocyte activity, increased natural killer cell number by 22-37%, with a 45% increase in killing ability.[6] If DHEA levels are found to be low through blood or salivary testing, starting at 5 mg a day is recommended and then slowly increased.

Growth Hormone

Growth hormone, or the "anti-aging" hormone, is secreted during sleep, which stimulates tissue regeneration, liver cleansing, muscle building, break down of fat stores and normalization of blood sugar.

Growth hormone and prolactin are required for the development of mature lymphocytes and to maintain immune action. These hormones help lymphocytes respond to invaders. Hormones and growth factors may all function as cytokines, the chemical messengers of the immune system.[7]

Estrogen, Testosterone, and Progesterone

Recent studies have clarified the interaction of estrogen and testosterone on the immune system in acute traumatic bleeding disorders. One study indicated testosterone levels depressed the immune system in trauma-hemorrhage, while estrogen seemed to exhibit immunoprotective properties by blocking any testosterone activity.[8]

Other studies demonstrate testosterone and estrogen are pro-inflammatory by stimulating certain immune cells.[9] Immune cells have specific receptors for estrogen and testosterone, suggesting a direct effect on immune system activity.[10] Progesterone strengthens the immune response indirectly by promoting growth hormone secretion during sleep.

Hormone Balancing

Because of the delicate balance between the hormonal system, nervous system, and immune system, hormonal support should only be given if there is a documented deficiency by a blood or saliva hormone test. Talk to your physician or natural health care provider regarding hormone testing and proper supplementation through herbs and bio-identical hormone replacement.

Help the Defense Team During Cold and Flu Season By Decreasing Exposure to Bacteria and Viruses

- Avoid people with colds when possible
- Wash your hands often. You can pick up cold germs easily, even when shaking someone's hand or touching doorknobs, handrails, toilet handles, gym equipment, gas pumps, shopping carts, or used tissue.
- Sneeze or cough into a tissue and then throw the tissue away and wash your hands to prevent transmission to others.
- Clean surfaces you touch with a germ-killing disinfectant such as tea tree oil, grapefruit seed extract, 1 in 10 bleach solution, or 70% isopropyl alcohol. Surfaces cleaned with bleach should remain wet for at least 10 minutes to be effective.
- Don't touch your nose, eyes, or mouth. Germs can enter your body easily by these paths.

- Use air filters at work and at home. Hepa air filters filter out 99% of air pollution including bacteria and viruses usually down to 0.3 microns in size. Purchasing air filters you can program to start and end at specific times are convenient to ensure a bedroom or office is filtered by the time you need to be in that space. Use special hepa furnace filters to decrease air pollution in your home.

---

[1] Gelfand, EW et al. (2003). The hygiene hypothesis revisited: Pros and cons. 60th Anniversary Meeting of the *American Academy of Allergy, Asthma and Immunology*.

2 Wiegert DA, Blalock JE. (1987). Interactions between the neuroendocrine and immune systems: common hormones and receptors. *Immunological Review*, 100:79-108.

[3] Wang, HC, and Klein, JR. (2001).Immune function of thyroid stimulating hormone and receptor. *Critical Review of Immunology*, 21(4): 323-37.

[4] Dickstein JB, Moldofsky H. (1999). Sleep, cytokines and immune function. *Sleep Medicine Review*, 3(3):219-28.

[5] Dorshkind, K and Horseman, ND. (2000). The roles of prolactin, growth hormone, insulin-like growth factor-I, and thyroid hormones in lymphocyte development and function: insights from genetic models of hormone and hormone receptor deficiency. *Endocrine Reviews*. 21(3): 292-312.

[6] Khorram, O. Vu, L, Yen, SS. (1997). Activation of immune function by dehydroepiandrosterone (DHEA) in age-advanced men. *Journal of Gerontology*, 52(1):M1-7.

[7] Berczi, I. (1997). Pituitary hormones and immune function. *Acta Paediatrica Suppl*, 423:70-5.

[8] Angele, MK, Schwacha, MG, Ayala, A, Chaudry, IH. (2000)Effect of gender and sex hormones on immune responses following shock. *Shock*, 14(2):81-90.

[9] Janele, D. et al. (2006). Effects of testosterone, 17beta-estradiol, and downstream estrogens on cytokine secretion from human leukocytes in the presence and absence of cortisol. *Annals of the New York Academy of Sciences,* 1069:168-82

[10] Angele, MK, Schwacha, MG, Ayala, A, Chaudry, IH. (2000)Effect of gender and sex hormones on immune responses following shock. *Shock*, 14(2):81-90.

3 | Immune Suppressive Activities

Immune suppressive activities are the leading culprits that weaken the immune system and leave it susceptible to most bacteria or viruses. The good news is that they are all habits that can be changed.

Top 10 Immune Suppressive Activities

Overdosing on sugar

Excess Alcohol or Smoking

Sleep Deprivation

Stress and Negative Emotions

Food Allergens

Being Overweight

Intense Prolonged Exercise or "Weekend Warrior"

Exposure to Pollution and Toxins

Structural Misalignment (Vertebral Subluxation)

Dehydration or Inadequate Nutrition

Do any of these sound familiar? This Top 10 list often answers the question "Why did I get sick?" Many people get sick at the start of a new school term, at Halloween, Thanksgiving, Christmas, and New Year's. However, by eliminating one or more immune suppressive activities, you can support your immune system and break the cycle of chronic colds and flus. To see how your lifestyle affects your immune system, take the Total Immune Suppression Test at the end of this chapter.

Sugar and the Immune System

Eating or drinking 100 grams (approximately 3 1/2 oz.) of sugar, glucose, fructose, honey, the equivalent of one 12-ounce can of soda, can reduce by 40% the ability of white blood cells to kill germs. The immune-suppressing effect of sugar starts less than thirty minutes after ingestion and may last for up to five hours.[1] In contrast, the ingestion of complex carbohydrates or starches which the body then converts to sugars has little or no effect on the immune system because the fiber slows down the conversion of starches to sugar in the body.

In addition to its effect on the immune system, high sugar intake has been implicated in poor memory (by shrinking areas in the brain), hypertension, obesity, diabetes, cancer, high cholesterol, hyperactivity, and anxiety, just to name a few.

Common Sources of Sugar

Unsweetened fruit juice: 30g per 8 oz.
Dried fruit: 29g per ¼ cup (raisins)
Yogurt: 20g per 6 oz. (vanilla)
Ice cream: 26g per 1/2 cup
Breakfast cereals: 13-20g per ½ cup
Toaster Pastries: 30g per 2 tarts
Pure Maple Syrup: 56g per 1/4 c

To better monitor sugar intake, read labels carefully for portion size and sugar content. If the words *sucrose, glucose, lactose, fructose, corn syrup, high fructose corn syrup,* or *white grape juice* appear on the label, sugar has been added to the product.

Sugar Reducing Tips

- Dilute fruit juice by 1/2 to 2/3 with water or carbonated water to cut sugar by over 50%.
- Buy plain yogurt and sweeten with frozen berries or stevia or mix 1/2 plain yogurt and 1/2 sweetened yogurt.
- Use alternative sweeteners, such as stevia or xylitol, instead of sugar to sweeten food.
- Avoid "white" or simple carbohydrates such as white rice, white flour, white potatoes as these turn into sugar quickly after ingesting and do not have the fiber to slow their absorption.
- Limit portions of sugary foods. For example, eat 2-3 small sugar cookies (about 5-12g of sugar instead of eating half the bag) could add up to 30-40g.

What About Alternative Sweeteners?

There are many so called "natural sweeteners" on the market. Calling something a "natural" sweetener does not mean it has less sugar than other sweeteners. Many products boast a natural sweetener but they contain fruit juice or brown rice syrup. These sweeteners quickly raise blood glucose and act similarly to sugar. However, stevia and sugar alcohols (such as xylitol) provide a sweet taste

with dramatically less sugar to suppress your immune
system or raise your blood sugar.

Stevia

Stevia is an extremely sweet herb, but it does not affect
blood sugar. Stevia leaves are ground and used to sweeten
many products, particularly in Japan and Paraguay. Stevia
stimulates sweet receptors on the tongue but is not
considered a sugar. Stevia has no calories, no
carbohydrates, protein, or fat. It is significantly sweeter
than sugar. Stevia has been shown in studies to prevent
pancreatic degeneration in people with diabetes and acts as
an immune regulator.[2] Stevia also has anti-inflammatory
and anti-cancer activity. However, a little goes a long way.
If you use too much stevia, you might experience an
unpleasant aftertaste. Stevia is sold in single serving
packets as well as in a liquid form. Liquid stevia can be
added drop by drop to avoid the aftertaste.

Sugar Alcohols

Sugar alcohols are carbohydrates that partially resemble
sugar and partially resemble alcohol, but they don't contain
ethanol, as alcoholic beverages do. Sugar alcohols are not
absorbed completely and thus contain fewer calories and
can sweeten foods without significantly increasing blood
sugar. They are found in sugar-free and reduced-sugar
products for individuals with diabetes, and in new products
developed for carbohydrate controlled eating plans.[3]

The most common sugar alcohols include sorbitol, mannitol, xylitol, maltitol, maltitol syrup, lactitol, erythritol, and isomalt. They contain 1-2.5 (36-67%) fewer calories per gram than sucrose (table sugar). Most are approximately half as sweet as sucrose, while maltitol and xylitol are about as sweet as sucrose.

Sugar alcohols occur naturally in fruits and vegetables, but are commercially produced from other carbohydrates such as sucrose, glucose, and starch. Sugar alcohols provide bulk in baking and moisture retention similar to sugar.

One sugar alcohol, xylitol, is derived from corn or birch trees. You may have heard of xylitol at your dentist's office as it has been shown to prevent oral bacterial growth, decreasing tooth decay and helping prevent ear infections in children.[4] One study demonstrated a 40% reduction in ear infections in children who chewed xylitol sweetened gum.[5]

Sugar alcohols can cause diarrhea, excess gas and other digestive problems in sensitive individuals or if ingested in large quantities. It is best to test their use in small amounts to see if they are well tolerated.

Honey
Although excessive amounts of honey can suppress the immune system, honey has been used for hundreds of years to fight skin infections and improve wound healing. Honey has antibacterial, antifungal, and antioxidants activities that

make it ideal for treating wounds. Research using Manuka honey, a honey made from bees gathering pollen from the flowers of the Manuka bush in New Zealand, have consistently shown anti-bacterial effects against most strains of bacteria including antibiotic resistant strains (MRSA, MSSA, and VRE). The study went on to cite synergistic effects of using honey and antibiotics together for wound healing.[6]

In addition to its wound healing effects, eating local honey could decrease seasonal allergies. Local honey contains pollen picked up from bees and introduces a small amount into your system. Ingesting small amounts of allergens helps desensitize your immune system to local pollen. If you have a severe or anaphylactic reaction to any food, animal or plant or suspect that you have leaky gut syndrome, oral desensitization is contraindicated. Typical recommendation is a teaspoon of local honey per day starting a few months prior to the pollen season to give your body a chance to lower its reaction to local pollens. Only local honey will work because it contains the pollens that are in your area.

Using Honey When Sick

The composition of honey makes it a natural expectorant (increases mucus clearing) and its anti-bacteria, antiviral effects on the mucus membranes of the mouth and upper throat make honey an ideal part of treating colds and flus for children over 12 months old.

In a comparison of 105 children with upper respiratory tract infections honey was rated more favorably than DM (Dextromethorphan) for symptomatic relief of nighttime cough and sleep difficulties due to the upper respiratory congestion.[7] Many herbal cough elixirs use honey to sweeten and for its own healing abilities.

Agave Nectar

Agave nectar is a natural fructose sweetener extracted from the Agave plant. It is about 1.4 times sweeter than regular sugar. Agave was once a go-to for alternative natural sweeteners because it has a 54% lower glycemic index (the higher a glycemic index food number is, the faster it raises your blood sugar level) than regular sugar. Now researchers know that it contains more fructose than high-fructose corn syrup. High levels of fructose are linked to increasing appetite and increased weight gain, especially belly fat, and can lead to insulin resistance. At this time nutritionists agree that agave should be avoided as a preferred sweetener although it is healthier than using artificial sweeteners.

Artificial Sweeteners

Artificial sweeteners are synthetic chemicals which create a sweet taste without affecting blood glucose and with significantly fewer calories than sugar. However, aspartame (NutraSweet, Equal) a popular artificial sweetener, has been implicated in an increased rate of lymphoma, leukemia, transitional cell carcinoma of the bladder, cervical dysplasia, and cancer of peripheral nerves in rats at doses less than the current acceptable daily intake.[8]

Since FDA approval, the Center for Disease Control has received numerous adverse reaction complaints against aspartame including altered brain function, behavior changes, fibromyalgia symptoms, multiple sclerosis symptoms, dizziness, headaches, and menstrual problems.[9]

Sucralose (Splenda), another artificial sweetener, can trigger migraine headaches in sensitive individuals.[10] Sucralose also increased insulin levels by 20% when combined with sucrose in overweight people. The artificial sweetener was related to an enhanced blood insulin and glucose response. Over time, higher levels of insulin can contribute to Type 2 diabetes.[11]

There is not enough evidence of safety to recommend artificial sweeteners at this time, as more natural alternatives with little to no side effects are available.

Sweetener Reminders
- Stevia and sugar alcohols sweeten, but will not activate yeast, so they are not a suitable sugar replacement in yeast-raised goods.
- Honey will activate yeast, but it does increase blood sugar.
- Alternative sweeteners are much sweeter than sugar. Each product has its own sugar conversion chart. For example, 1/3 tsp to 1 tsp of stevia = 1 c sugar.

- Substituting the right amount of alternative sweeteners is important as too much can cause diarrhea or an unpleasant after taste.
- Artificial sweeteners may have significant side effects and generally should be avoided.

Excess Alcohol and the Immune System

Alcohol intake interferes with a variety of immune defenses. Research indicates excessive alcohol consumption is linked with certain types of cancers and infections. Excessive alcohol consumption produces an overall nutritional deficiency, depriving the body of valuable immune-boosting nutrients. Alcohol intake affects the digestion, storage, utilization, and excretion of many important vitamins and minerals especially vitamin A, C, D, E, K and B vitamins.[12] Alcohol, like sugar, consumed in excess can reduce the ability of white blood cells to kill germs. Alcohol also causes a dysregulation of blood sugar causing low or excessive amounts in the blood contributing to immune suppression.

Excess alcohol is defined as three or more drinks in most research studies. One drink does not suppress the immune system. In fact, a moderate amount of red wine (1-2 glasses a day) does not decrease immune function and helps protect against heart disease.[13] Individual response to alcohol varies depending on tolerance levels. Immune suppression is likely if one drinks enough to feel intoxicated even if it is under three drinks.

Cigarettes and the Immune System

Cigarette smoke either inhaled directly or second hand is saturated with toxic chemicals, most of which negatively impact immune response. Cigarette smoke actually causes T lymphocyte cell death and interferes with immune cell maturation in unborn children of smoking mothers.[14]

Cigarette smoke, either first or second hand, is also an irritant to mucous membranes of the body, namely the lungs, throat, nose, and ear mucosa, predisposing these areas to infection.

Sleep and Immune Function

Getting enough sleep is essential for a healthy immune system. When we sleep, the immune system is replenished. Even one night's sleep loss can significantly suppress the immune system. Studies on people suffering from insomnia (problems in falling or staying asleep) have identified fatigue, immunodepression, weight gain, irritability, depression, and memory issues directly related to not getting enough sleep.[15] Most of these are due to a deficiency of growth hormone produced while we sleep.

Sleep studies have shown significant changes in immune function due to the interaction of prolactin, growth hormone, and cortisol during sleep. Even one night of 5 hours sleep deprivation from 10 pm to 3 am depressed natural killer cells and T cells.[16] Growth hormone is needed to maintain mature T cells and a variety of other functions in the body. (See *Hormone* section in *Meet the Defense Team* for more information).

Studies examining sleep and weight gain have identified significant risk factors for obesity if sleeping 5 or less hours a night. Sleeping 5 hours a night increased the likelihood of obesity by 50%. Sleeping 4 or less hours a night increased the risk of obesity by 73%.[17] Most of these factors are due to changes in leptin and ghrelin, two hormones that affect eating patterns. With sleep deprivation leptin, a hormone that tells the body that it is full, is decreased. Ghrelin, a hormone that tells the body that it is hungry, is increased by 24%. Ghrelin also signals the body to crave starchy, sweet foods. The combination of increased appetite (ghrelin) and decreased sense of fullness (leptin) along with growth hormone effects on insulin and fat deposits creates a prime environment for weight gain or difficulty losing weight.

In other studies, 5-10 days of sleep deprivation (acute or chronic lack of sufficient sleep i.e. less than recommended) decreased antioxidant levels in vital organs increasing the risk for chronic disease and cancer.[18] Being sleep deprived also increases the risk and severity of depression, ADHD/ADD, decreases one's ability to handle stress and affects one's ability to remember facts and think clearly.[19]

Many of these factors affect teens the most since they are most often sleep deprived due to a change in sleep-wake cycles due to puberty. Most teens find that they cannot fall asleep until 11 or 12 am and then wake up for school at 5:30 or 6:00 am leaving them with 5.5 to 7 hours of sleep a night (8.5-9.25 hours is recommended). The sleep debt that is caused by this schedule cannot be made up by sleeping in on the weekend. Specific supplements and light therapy can correct most teen sleep problems. Talk to your naturopathic doctor or pediatrician for specific recommendations.

The National Sleep Foundation has provided general sleep recommendations listed below; however, individual requirements can vary so finding out how much sleep one needs to feel rested and at peak performance is important. Living at a higher altitude generally requires an additional hour of sleep compared to a lower altitude.

2015 National Sleep Foundation Recommendations[20]	
Newborns (0-3 months)	14-17 hours
Infants (4-11 months)	12-15 hours
Toddlers (1-2 years)	11-14 hours
Preschool (3-5 years)	10-13 hours
School Age (6-13 years)	9-11 hours
Teens (14-17 years)	8-10 hours
Young Adults (18-25)	7-9 hours
Adults and Older Adults	7-9 hours
Older Adults (65+)	7-8 hours

Stress and the Immune System

Keeping stress under control is essential for a healthy immune system. When we are stressed, our adrenal glands secrete a hormone known as cortisol. Although cortisol is helpful to keep inflammation in check, overproduction on an ongoing basis can create problems.

For example, when cortisol output is high, the immune system secretes interleukin 6 (IL-6), which contributes to inflammation. IL-6 is also believed to cause autoimmune diseases such as rheumatoid arthritis and fibromyalgia to worsen, to cause calcium to leave the bones, and to act as a growth factor for a number of tumors.

Emotional/Social Stress and the Immune System

Five minutes of strong negative emotions, such as anger, can knock down the immune system for up to 6 hours. Researchers determined this by measuring levels of immune protecting chemicals in saliva. According to the International College of Integrative Medicine, "It takes 6 hours for salivary IgA to return to baseline after only five minutes of anger."[21]

Therefore, just 20 minutes of strong negative emotion suppresses the immune system for one entire day. Happiness, on the other hand, increases immune cells (specifically IgA) and decreases cortisol, a substance secreted in higher quantities during stress which suppresses the immune system. It seems individuals who frequently experience negative emotions have a slower immune response and may be at risk for illness, more so than those who frequently experience positive emotions.

A specific type of response to stress and emotions has been identified in many cancer patients. Psychologists call this pattern the "Type C" or biopsychosocial cancer risk pattern. The common patterns noted are denial and suppression of emotions (in particular anger), "pathological niceness," avoidance of conflicts, exaggerated social desirability, harmonizing behavior, over-compliance, over-patience, as well as high rationality and a rigid control of emotional expression.[22] A prominent feature of this particular coping style (excessive denial, avoidance, suppression of emotions and one's own basic needs) appears to weaken the body's natural resistance to cancer-causing influences. This coping style is associated with immune suppression in many areas of the immune system.

Stress Reduction Techniques

Stress affects the immune system, whether it be physical (see *Intense Prolonged Exercise* section), mental or emotional. The effects of stress on immune function are profound and long lasting. Cultivating ways of reducing stress through deep breathing, exercise, prayer, meditation, a positive outlook on life, journaling, guided imagery, biofeedback, or just talking with a friend or loved one are all effective ways to reduce the negative impact of stress on your immune system.

Stress happens! How we respond to stress is our choice and that choice affects the immune system. Healthy responses to stress involve a sense of control over health and quality of life, a strong commitment to work, creative activities or relationships, and an ability to see stress as a challenge rather than a threat.[23]

Food Allergies and the Immune System

Since over 50% of the immune system resides in the digestive tract, digestive tract health is paramount for a strong immune system. Food allergies or immune-mediated food reactions can "wear out the immune system." Because the immune system is constantly fighting the "allergic" foods, it doesn't have the reserves it needs when an actual virus or bacteria is present.

Common Signs of Food Allergies

- Eczema, rashes around the mouth, anus, behind ears, around nose, hives, dark circles under the eyes, acne
- Indigestion, nausea, vomiting, irritable bowel syndrome, diarrhea, constipation, gas, bloating, stomach ulcers, pruritus ani, cramping pain, ulcerative colitis, Crohn's disease, colic (in babies), gall bladder disease
- Chronic runny/stuffy nose, chronic sinus infections, chronic colds
- Muscle aches, osteoarthritis, rheumatoid arthritis, fibromyalgia

• Mood swings, anxiety, depression, food cravings, poor
concentration, fatigue, hyperactivity, cranky behavior in
children
• Fatigue, headaches, high blood pressure, arrhythmia,
angina
• Frequent urination, burning with urination, bedwetting in
children

Food Introduction in Infants

Thoughtful food introduction is important to prevent and
identify food allergies in infants. Thoughtful food
introduction involves introducing one food at a time,
waiting three days to see if there is an adverse reaction and,
finally, waiting to introduce highly allergenic foods until
the child is at least 1-1/2 years old. Highly allergenic foods
include eggs, soy, wheat, dairy, peanuts, corn, and shellfish.

Testing For Food Allergies

There are many different tests that can identify food
allergies. Some test for immediate food reactions while
others include testing for delayed allergic reactions. Talk
to your doctor about which test is best for you:

- Blood test
- Skin testing (scratch or prick tests)
- RAST test
- Allergy Elimination Diet
- Pulse test

Mucous Producing Foods

Some foods stimulate mucous production and suppress immune function by causing congestion. Congestion decreases blood flow causing decreased access to the area by immune cells and decreased waste removal thus increasing the "food" available for bacteria/viruses. These are not food allergies per se but rather a physiological reaction. Avoiding the following mucous producing foods during a cold/flu can decrease the duration of the illness: dairy products, oranges, and bananas.

Overweight

Being overweight can lead to a depressed immune system by affecting the ability of white blood cells to multiply, produce antibodies, and rush to the site of an infection due to decreased blood flow to areas of the body.[24] Being overweight also contributes to blood sugar dysregulation which can increase susceptibility to infection, decrease memory, and lead to poor wound healing. Blood sugar dysregulation is caused by insensitivity in the control system affecting cortisol.[25]

Intense Prolonged Exercise

Exercise is a wonderful immune booster and good for virtually every part of you! A program of regular, moderate exercise relieves stress and makes it easier for you to sleep at night. Exercise has been shown to reverse part of the age-related decline in immune functioning.[26]

In general, exercising less than 60 minutes at less than 60% intensity causes the least amount of stress to the immune system. Running a marathon or performing any other activity that is intense and continues for over 4-5 hours actually suppresses immune activity. Various studies demonstrate neutrophil activity suppression with intense prolonged exercise.[27] Because neutrophils are the major immune cell that attacks bacteria, upper respiratory tract infections are reported more often in athletes involved in intense prolonged exercise. The only immune cells elevated in high-performance athletes are NK cells. NK cells are involved in searching out bacteria, viruses, and precancerous cells.

Other factors beyond exercise-specific immune suppression (such as mental stress, undernourishment, quick weight loss, and improper hygiene) have each been associated with impaired immunity in athletes who are undergoing heavy training regimens.[28]

Should I Exercise When I Am Sick?

With infections, the body uses all of its energy reserves to fight off invaders. It is important to not physically fatigue the body during this time. A quick guideline is to exercise to the point you could do the same routine two to three more times without becoming exhausted.

Clinical case studies and animal data suggest infection severity, relapse, and myocarditis (inflammation of the heart muscle) may result when patients exercise vigorously while sick.[29] However, mild exercise can increase blood flow and stimulate the immune system.

Pollution/Toxins

Pollution is a major factor in immune suppression. In a Russian study, pollution contributed to significant immune suppression and damage to the immune system. Unfortunately, toxic chemicals are everywhere around us. Learning to recognize harmful chemicals in the home and outside environment can help you decrease your exposure.

According to the Environmental Protection Agency, indoor pollution is more of a health issue than outdoor pollution. Indoor pollution comes primarily from volatile organic chemicals (VOC) like formaldehyde, present in new building materials such as carpeting, paneling, cabinets, fabrics, etc. Other sources come from cleaning fluids, sprays, fumes from copiers/faxes or in plug in air fresheners.

Ways to Decrease Indoor Pollution
- Buy (or make) non-toxic cleaning fluids/sprays
- Use baking soda instead of commercial powder cleansers to clean the bathroom
- Use vinegar to clean windows
- Use tea tree oil to kill mold and mildew
- Use live enzyme cultures (such as Biokleen brand cleaners) to break up soap residue and stains
- Leave shoes at the door to reduce tracked-in lead, dust, and pesticides by a factor of 10-20

- Use a hepa air filter (at work and at home) to clean the air of toxins with the added benefit of filtering out airborne viruses/bacteria. Use a central vacuuming apparatus or hepa vacuum to help to minimize pollutants in the air
- Filter all public water to remove toxic particles, chemicals, heavy metals, and microorganisms
- Install full spectrum lights to reduce eye-strain and increase UV absorption
- Reduce electromagnetic exposure from microwaves, electric blankets, ungrounded electrical outlets, and other electrical appliances (such as computers, cell phones, etc.) to keep your toxic exposure down
- Use essential oils and baking soda to reduce odor in the home instead of chemical air fresheners
- Add plants that promote clean air to your office and home. NASA has spent two decades researching plants that remove toxic chemicals from the air for use in space stations
- The following six plants have been found to be particularly effective in clearing the air of formaldehyde, benzene, and trichloroethylene:[30]

    Mass cane (Dracaena Massangeana)
    Pot mum (Chrysanthemum Morifolium)
    Gerbera daisy (Gerbera Jamesonii)
    Warnecki (Dracaena Deremensis "Warneckei")
    Ficus (Ficus Benjamina)
    Rubber tree (Ficus Elastica)

Most of these plants are poisonous when ingested. When children or pets are around, take care with the placement and accessibility of the plant.

Structural Misalignment/Vertebral Subluxation

A well-aligned spine is able to transmit nerve activity without restriction, thus supporting the immune system by providing it with important information. If there are areas of subluxation/misalignment, nerve and blood flow is impaired and since the immune system relies heavily on its communication and transport networks, it is impaired in its actions.

In addition to nerve and blood flow issues, specific vertebrae (such as C1) can rotate out of alignment and compress the Eustachian tube, contributing to ear infections and other upper respiratory infections. Upper back misalignment (especially at T5-T8) can impair the function of the lungs to clear mucus from the airways and increases the risk of infection in the airways.

Getting regular care for your spine, making your work space ergonomic and exercising/stretching regularly are key to improving immune system efficiency and spinal health. Pilates and yoga are also excellent exercises to strengthen and tone your spine and provide immune stimulation when performed in moderation.

Dehydration and Inadequate Nutrition

Over 75% of the body is comprised of water. The body relies on fluids for cellular communication, transportation of nutrients, immune cells, oxygen, proteins, and hormones. When we are dehydrated, immune cells are not able to get to sites where they are needed, increasing infections and inflammation.

Dehydration is a common occurrence for the typical American, especially at high altitudes. Dehydration occurs when water intake is less than water output. Caffeine and stress both contribute to excess water loss.

Laboratory tests to check red blood cell values can confirm dehydration. Most annual physical blood tests will check these parameters. Looking at an optimal range of red blood cell values easily confirms dehydration. Most patients that I evaluate are moderately to significantly dehydrated on review of blood tests.

How much water should I drink?

A simple way to stay hydrated is to drink 1/2 of your body weight in ounces per day. For example, a 120 lb. person should drink 60 oz. of water a day. An additional 8 oz. of water should be consumed for each cup of caffeinated beverage and for each hour of exercise. If a 120 lb. person actively worked for 3 hours and drank 8oz of coffee and a glass of ice tea in the afternoon, their total water intake should be 60+24+16=100 oz. a day.

People who suffer from kidney disease, congestive heart failure or who take diuretic medication or other electrolyte dependent medications should speak with their physician before significantly changing water intake.

Inadequate Nutrition

Inadequate nutrition is commonly seen with the typical American diet consisting largely of processed and fast foods. Processed and fast foods are much lower in certain vitamins and minerals that are crucial for the immune system. Most Americans are overfed and undernourished creating major problems for the immune system and overall health (see Chapter 3 *Immune Supportive Diet* for more details).

Total Immune Suppression Test

Take the test and see how your lifestyle rates. The test is modified from Holmes and Rahe Social Adjustment Scale and Total Life Stress Test.[31,32]

Check the answers appropriate for you.

Sugar Consumption (per day)   (total used)
| | |
Sugar added to food or drink (teaspoons)   0 1 2 3 4
Sweet roll, pie/cake piece, brownie or other dessert   0 1 2 3 4
Soda, candy bar or 8 oz. fruit juice   0 1 2 3 4
Ice cream ½ cup   0 1 2 3 4
White bread / white rice/ pasta (1 serving)   0 1 2 3 4

Subtotal_____ x 10 = ____

Alcohol Consumption

1 drink= 1 oz. whiskey, gin or vodka, 8 oz. beer or 4-6 oz. wine

2-3 drinks per day	4
3 or more drinks per day	10
Drinking to intoxication	15

Subtotal_____

Cigarette Smoke

Exposed to second-hand cigarette smoke more than 1 hour per day	4
Smoke 3-10 cigarettes per day	4
Smoke 11-20 cigarettes per day	8
Smoke 21-30 cigarettes per day	10
Smoke 31-40 cigarettes per day	20
Smoke over 40 cigarettes per day	40
Smoke cigars once or twice a day	4
Smoke a pipe once or twice a day	4
Use chewing tobacco once or twice a day	8

Subtotal_____

Sleep

Sleep less than 5 hours one night a week	10
Sleeps less than 7 hours a night 3 or more nights a week	20
Wakes from sleep 2-3 times a night for more than 10 min	10

Subtotal_____

Stress

Work stress

Work more than 50 hours per week	10
Work varying shifts	10
Work night shift	10
Frustration at work	4
Boss doesn't trust me	8
Lack of authority at work	8

Social Stress

Divorce	7
Personal injury or illness	5
Change in financial status	4
Death of a close family member	5
Retirement	5
Trouble with boss on a social level	3
Change in school, recreation, church activities, or work hours	4

Emotions (most days of the week)

Moderately angry, depressed, or frustrated	10
Very angry, depressed, or frustrated	20

(0 =agree 4= completely disagree)

Believe I am responsible for my happiness	0 1 2 3 4
Satisfied and in control of my life	0 1 2 3 4
Any other major emotional stress not mentioned	
(1-10 intensity)	_____

Subtotal_____

Overweight

10-16 lb. overweight	5
16-25 lb. overweight	10
26-40 lb. overweight	20
More than 40 lb. overweight	40

Subtotal_____

Physical Activity

30 min of exercise 3 or more days per week	-20
Some physical activity, 1-2 days a week	-5
No regular exercise	25
Intense physical exercise, over 4-5 hours per day	30
Subtotal	

Pollution Indoor and Outdoor

Live within 10 miles of a city of 500,000 or more	4
Live within 10 miles of a city of 250,000 or more	2
Live within 10 miles of a city of 50,000 or more	2
Live in the country but use pesticide, herbicide and /or chemical fertilizer	4
Live in a home built in the last two years	4
New paint, carpets, or furniture	3
Live in a pre-fabricated home built in the last two years	5
Work in an office with recycled air	3
Work with paints, toner, or other chemicals	5
Subtotal	

Structural Misalignment

Pain when vertebrae are touched	10
Neck or back pain 2 to 3 times a week	5
Chronic low back or neck pain most days of the week	15
Work involves heavy labor when not physically fit	20
Work at a non- ergonomic desk	15
Subtotal	

Dehydration/ Poor Nutrition

Drink 5 or less 16 oz. glasses of water a day	5
Drink less than 2 16 oz. glasses of water a day	15
Drink more than one caffeinated beverage a day (coffee, tea, soda)	5
One meal a day of processed foods/fast food restaurant (boxed or frozen pre-prepared meals)	5
Two meals a day of processed/fast food	10
All meals a day are from processed/fast food	25
Subtotal	

TOTAL SCORE_____

Review your total score and each individual category in order to identify major immune suppressive areas to improve upon.

10-25   Mild immune suppression likely
26-50   Moderate immune suppression likely
51-100   Severe immune suppression likely

[1] Sanchez A, et al. (1973). Role of sugars in human neutrophilic phagocytosis. *American Journal of Clinical Nutrition*, 26(11):1180-4.

[2] Boonkaewwan C, Toskulkao C, Vongsakul M. (2006). Anti-Inflammatory and Immunomodulatory Activities of Stevioside and Its Metabolite Steviol on THP-1 Cells. *Journal of Agriculture and Food Chemistry*, 8;54(3):785.

[3] International Food Information Council.(2004). Sugar alcohol fact sheet. http://http://www.ific.org/publications/factsheets/sugaralcoholfs.cfm

[4] Makinen, KK et al. (1995). Xylitol chewing gums and caries rates: a 40-month cohort study. *Journal of Dental Research*. 74: 1904-13.

[5] Niemela, M, Kontiokari, T and Uhari, M. (1998). A novel use of xylitol sugar in preventing acute otitis media. *Pediatrics*. 102: 879-84.

[6] Carter, D et al. (2016). Therapeutic Manuka Honey: No Longer So Alternative. Frontiers in Microbiology. 7: 569.

[7] Paul, IM, et al. (2007). Effect of Honey, Dextromethorphan, and No Treatment on Nocturnal Cough and Sleep Quality for Coughing Children and Their Parents. *Archives Pediatric Adolescent Medicine*. 161(12). 1140-1146.

[8] Belpoggi, F et al. (2006). First experimental demonstration of the multipotential carcinogenic effects of aspartame administered in the feed to Sprague-Dawley rats. *Environmental Health Perspectives.* 114, 379-85.

[9] Garriga, MM and Metcalfe, DD. (1988) Aspartame intolerance. *Annals of Allergy.* Dec;61:63-9.

[10] Grimsley, E, Patel, RM, Sarma, R. (2006). Popular sweetener Sucralose as a migraine trigger. *Annals of Allergy*,46(8):1303-4

[11] M. Yianna Pepion, Courtney D. Thiemann, Bruce W. Patterson, Burton M. Wace, Samuel Klein.(2013). Sucralose Affects Glycemic and Hormonal Responses to an Oral Glucose Load. *Diabetes Care.* Apr; DC_122221.

[12] National Institute on Alcohol Abuse and Alcoholism.(1993) Alcohol Alert. 22. PH 346.

[13] Watzl, B. et al. (2004). Daily moderate amounts of red wine or alcohol have no effect on the immune system of healthy men. *European Journal of Clinical Nutrition.* Jan;58(1):40-5.

[14] Kalra R, Singh SP, Savage SM, Finch GL, Sopori ML. (2000). Effects of cigarette smoke on immune response: chronic exposure to cigarette smoke impairs antigen-mediated signaling in T cells and depletes IP3-sensitive Ca(2+) stores. *Journal of Pharmacology and Experimental Therapeutics.*Apr;293(1):166-71.

[15] Anderson, RA. (2001). *Clinician's guide to holistic medicine.* Chicago: McGraw Hill.

[16] Irwin, M et al. (1996). Partial night sleep deprivation reduces natural killer and cellular immune responses in humans. *The FASEBJournal.* Apr 10(5):643-53.

[17] Emsellem, HA and Whiteley, C. (2006). *Snooze or Lose: No war ways to improve your teen's sleep habits.* Washington, DC: Joseph Henry Press.

[18] Emsellem, HA and Whiteley, C. (2006). *Snooze or Lose: No war ways to improve your teen's sleep habits.* Washington, DC: Joseph Henry Press.

[19] Emsellem, HA and Whiteley, C. (2006). *Snooze or Lose: No war ways to improve your teen's sleep habits.* Washington, DC: Joseph Henry Press.

[20] Retrieved 11/20/2016 from https://sleepfoundation.org/media-center/press-release/national-sleep-foundation-recommends-new-sleep-times.

[21] International College of Integrative Medicine. (2002) Chelation Therapy Workshop, March. Tampa Florida.

[22] Baltrusch HJ, Stangel W, Titze I. (1991). Stress, cancer and immunity. New developments in biopsychosocial and psychoneuroimmunologic research. *Acta neurologica.* Aug;13(4):315-27.

[23] Dreher, H. (1995). *The immune power personality.* New York: Dutton.

[24] Murray, MT. (1993). *The healing power of foods.* Rocklin, CA: Prima Publishing.

[25] Jessop, et al (2001). Resistance to glucocorticoid feedback in obesity. *Journal of Clinical Endocrinology and Metabolism.* 86: 4109–4114.

[26] Aria, MH, Duarte, AJ, and Natale, VM. (2006). The effects of long-term endurance training on the immune and endocrine systems of elderly men: the role of cytokines and anabolic hormones. *Immune Ageing.* Aug 25;3:9.

[27] Nieman, DC. (1997). Exercise immunology: practical applications. International Journal of Sports Medicine. Supp l 1:S91-100.

28 Nieman, DC. (1997). Exercise immunology: practical applications. International Journal of Sports Medicine. Supp l 1:S91-100.

[29] Nieman, DC. (1997). Exercise immunology: practical applications. *International Journal of Sports Medicine*. Supp 1 1:S91-100.

[30] Environmental Protection Agency. Plants That Promote Clean Air. www.epa.gov.

[31] Holmes, TH and Rahe, RH. The social readjustment rating scale. *Journal of Psychosomatic Research*, 11:213-213.

[32] Shealy, NC. (1999). *DHEA, the youth and health hormone*. Chicago: Keats.

4 | Immune Supportive Diet

The single most important thing we can do to support our immune system nutritionally and prevent most chronic diseases is to eat a balanced, organic, whole foods diet low in sugar. For most people, this means eating more whole fruits, vegetables, beans, nuts, and whole grains.

What are whole foods?

Whole foods are not refined, concentrated, or changed in any way prior to cooking. The refinement process in boxed foods or processed grains (such as white flour) depletes the food of important vitamins and minerals and degrades natural enzymes important for digesting food. A study examining the exact nutrient depletion of processed grains identified 50-90% depletion of important nutrients such as zinc, B vitamins, essential fatty acids, calcium, magnesium, and chromium.[1]

How can I tell if something is a whole food?

Ask yourself these questions:[2]

- Can I imagine it growing?
- How many ingredients does it have? A whole food just has one ingredient--itself.

- What has been done to the food since it was harvested?
  Pick the least processed food. Most processed foods don't
  resemble anything in nature. Read the labels; if you can't
  pronounce it, don't eat it.

Typically, grocery stores stock whole foods in the
perimeter aisles, so avoid the center aisles full of processed
foods.

Organic Foods

Organic farmers must grow crops without using most
conventional pesticides, petroleum-based fertilizers, or
sewage sludge-based fertilizers. Animals raised on an
organic operation must be fed organic feed and given
access to the outdoors. They are given no antibiotics or
growth hormones.[3]

Benefits of Organic Foods

Eating organic decreases your exposure to pesticides and
insecticides linked with many cancers. Pesticide residues
have been linked to promoting estrogen-sensitive cancers
(such as breast and uterine) and to childhood cancers (such
as leukemia and lymphoma).

Organic foods contain higher levels of many important
minerals such as calcium, magnesium, iron, and copper. In
addition, organic farming decreases chemical
contamination of water and land.

A recent study from Emory University in Atlanta
analyzed urine samples from children ages three to 11 who

ate only organic foods and found they contained virtually no metabolites of two common pesticides, malathion and chlorpyrifos. However, once the children returned to eating conventionally grown foods, concentrations of these pesticide metabolites quickly climbed as high as 263 parts per billion.[4]

Pesticides and Cancer

In women with breast cancer, pesticide levels have been shown to be at higher levels when compared with women with benign breast disease.[5]

Several studies link leukemia to pesticides. Two recent reviews concluded pesticide exposure may be a cause of leukemia.[6,7] These reviews report most (though not all) studies find leukemia was more likely in children whose fathers were exposed to pesticides at work than other children. Risks for children are often reported to be greater than risks for adults.[8]

One large recent study of 491 children with acute lymphocytic leukemia (ALL) found risk was increased by home use of some kinds of pesticides and by use of multiple different pesticides. Herbicide use during pregnancy was associated with a 50% increase in risk. Use of insecticides in the home was associated with increased risk of ALL and frequent use was associated with higher risk. Use of some garden products also seemed to increase risk. The heightened risk was associated with use of multiple products.[9]

What foods should I buy organic?

It is best if you can purchase all organic foods. However, if you have to choose, buy organic foods on the *Dirty Dozen* list and foods containing higher fat concentrations (such as meats, eggs, milk, cheese, nuts, seeds, and olive oil) since toxins accumulate more readily in the fat.

The *Dirty Dozen* is a group of foods with the highest levels of pesticides. Most of these are foods children love to eat, making the organic choice an important one for your child's health.

The Dirty Dozen[10]
(in alphabetical order)
  Apples
  Celery
  Cherries
  Cherry tomatoes
  Cucumber
  Nectarines
  Peaches
  Potatoes
  Spinach
  Strawberries
  Sweet bell peppers
  Tomatoes
  Kale, Collard greens, and hot peppers also came up high in pesticides but didn't make the top 10.

Protein and the Immune System

Your immune system needs protein to provide the building blocks for immune cells and antibody production.

Protein also helps transport nutrients in the blood, produce important hormones, and produce essential digestive enzymes.[11] It is important to eat some protein with every meal and snack to stabilize blood sugar and sustain your energy throughout the day.

Since animal protein is often loaded with arachadonic acid and saturated fat, it is crucial to select organic, health conscious sources of protein such as wild fish, poultry, lean pork, nuts, and beans.

Because of the high fat content of meat, it is important to consume organic meat to avoid pesticide residues concentrated in the fatty portion of the meat and to decrease your exposure to added growth hormones and antibiotics non-organic meat usually contains. Added growth hormone interferes with your body's natural hormone balance and has been linked to early puberty changes in young girls.

Protein RDA for Children
    Ages 1-3   25 grams a day
    Ages 4-6   30 grams a day

Protein Needs for Adults
    Protein needs for adults are calculated based on weight (0.36 grams/lb.). For most people protein needs range from 40-70 grams a day.
    For example a person weighing 140 lb. should consume 50.4 grams of protein a day.

Food Sources of Protein

    Almonds: 7.3 g per ¼ cup
    Beef: 22 g per 3 oz.
    Broccoli: 8 g per 1 cup cooked
    Cheese: 11g per 1.5 oz.
    Cottage cheese: 20.5 g per 2/3 cup
    Chicken: 26 g per 3 oz.
    Whole wheat pasta: 10 g per 3/4 cup
    Black beans: 15 g per 1 cup cooked
    Clams: 65 g per 3 oz.
    Kidney beans: 18 g per 1 cup
    White fish: 17 g per 3oz
    Crabmeat: 42 g per 1 cup

Simple Protein Snacks to Keep You Going

    Whole grain toast with nut butter (almond, cashew,
        peanut)
    Protein shake with fresh fruit added
    Fresh or dried fruit (unsulphured only) with raw nuts
    Vegetable sticks with cheese or nut butter (almond,
        cashew, or peanut)
    Hard-boiled egg
    Hummus on whole grain crackers or with carrots,
        celery, cucumbers
    Apple and pear slices with nut butter
    Low-fat cottage cheese
    Bean dip with tortilla chips

Vitamins for Immune Health

Vitamin A and Beta carotene

Beta carotene increases the number of infection-fighting cells, natural killer cells, and helper T-cells and as a powerful antioxidant it mops up excess free radicals which accelerate aging.

Beta carotene also protects against cancer by stimulating macrophage immune cells to produce tumor necrosis factor, which kills cancer cells. It has also been shown beta carotene supplements can increase the production of T-cell lymphocytes and natural killer cells and can enhance the ability of the natural killer cells to attack cancer cells.

The body converts beta carotene to vitamin A, which itself has anticancer properties and immune-boosting functions. Conversion of beta carotene to vitamin A requires zinc, proper thyroid hormone levels, and vitamin C. If your body has adequate levels of vitamin A, it knows how to store beta carotene and not convert it to vitamin A. Too much vitamin A can be toxic to your body, so it's better to get extra beta carotene from foods and let the body naturally regulate how much of this precursor is converted to the immune-fighting vitamin A.

Food sources of Beta carotene and Vitamin A
Carrot juice: 250,000 IU per cup
Cod liver oil: 14,000 IU per Tb

Burdock/yellow dock steamed: 12,900 IU per cup
Sweet potato: 12,000 IU per medium potato
Spinach: 7,300 IU per ½ cup steamed
Collard greens/kale: 4500-5000 IU ½ cup steamed.

Vitamin C

There has been more research about the immune-boosting effects of vitamin C than perhaps any other nutrient.

Vitamin C increases the production of infection-fighting white blood cells and antibodies and increases levels of interferon (the antibody that coats cell surfaces, preventing the entry of viruses). As an added perk, people whose diets are higher in vitamin C have lower rates of colon, prostate, and breast cancer.

If you take vitamin C supplements, it's best to space doses throughout the day rather than taking one large dose, most of which may end up being excreted in the urine.

During an infection or at the beginning of an illness you can take vitamin C to bowel tolerance (the highest dose that doesn't cause diarrhea). Often amounts as high as 6000-7000 mg a day can be tolerated when you are sick without causing diarrhea. Vitamin C supplements with bioflavonoids increase vitamin C's action. If the acidic quality of vitamin C bothers your stomach, choose a buffered form.

Food Sources of Vitamin C
    Orange juice: 124 mg per cup
    Guava: 110 mg per cup
    Red chili pepper: 109 mg per medium pepper
    Green pepper: 94 mg per medium pepper
    Grapefruit: 82 mg per grapefruit

Choose low-sugar sources of vitamin C, as sugar will negate the effects of vitamin C. Chewable vitamin C should also be avoided because it creates an acidic environment in the mouth that can deteriorate enamel on teeth and is usually high in sugar. For those that cannot swallow pills (small children), powdered vitamin C is the best source followed by water to rinse out the mouth.

Vitamin D

Vitamin D, calciferol, is a fat-soluble vitamin found in food and made in your body after exposure to ultraviolet rays from the sun. Vitamin D boosts bacteria killing white blood cells (macrophages) and enhances the body's natural antibiotic molecules within the respiratory tract. Studies have shown that vitamin D reduces the frequency of respiratory infections in children. Some researchers have hypothesized that the flu is a symptom of vitamin D deficiency, but more research is needed to prove this.

Vitamin D helps to balance an overactive immune response as in autoimmune conditions. Vitamin D receptors are located on B cells, T cells and antigen presenting cells. Deficiency in vitamin D is associated with increased autoimmunity as well as an increased susceptibility to infection.[12]

Currently, 2000 IU a day is recommended to combat cold and flu and boost the immune system. Vitamin D accumulates in the body over time. Get blood tested to check vitamin D levels to identify a deficiency and the need to supplement in higher amounts.

Symptoms that may indicate a vitamin D deficiency are thin, brittle, soft, or misshapen bones, muscle weakness, feeling of heaviness in the legs, chronic musculoskeletal pain, fatigue or easy tiring, frequent infections, depression(general or seasonal).

Other conditions commonly treated with vitamin D
    Arthritis
    Autoimmune Disorders
    Cancer (Breast, Prostate, Colon and Skin)
    Chronic pain
    Cardiovascular health
    Depression and Seasonal Affective Disorder
    Diabetes
    Fatigue
    Infertility and PMS
    Obesity
    Osteoporosis
    Syndrome X

Sources of Vitamin D

Food sources: Cod liver oil, salmon, mackerel, tuna, sardines, fortified foods (milk, cereal, and margarine), eggs, beef liver, and Swiss cheese. Most contain less than 300 IU per serving. In general, food sources are not high enough in vitamin D to offer adequate amounts without sun exposure or supplementation.

Exposure to Sunlight: UV rays from sunlight triggers vitamin D synthesis in skin. Up to 20,000 IU can be synthesized by direct sun exposure. Season, latitude, time of day, cloud cover, smog, and sunscreens affect UV ray exposure. For example, in Boston the average amount of sunlight is insufficient to produce significant vitamin D synthesis in the skin from November through February. Tanning beds are also a source of UV rays and if used sparingly can significantly increase vitamin D levels. Care should be taken to limit time to 25% to 50% of the time it would take for the skin to turn a light pink and only go three times a week. **Sunscreens with a sun protection factor of 8 or greater will block UV rays that produce vitamin D.**

Calculate sun exposure to receive 5000 IU a day. Visit http://nadir.nilu.no/~olaeng/fastrt/VitD-ez_quartMED.html to calculate your specific sun time. You will need the latitude and longitude of your city.

Vitamin E

Vitamin E stimulates the production of natural killer cells which seek out and destroy germs and cancer cells. Vitamin E enhances the production of B-cells, the immune cells that produce antibodies to destroy bacteria. Vitamin E supplementation may also reverse some of the decline in immune response commonly seen in aging.

You need 100-400 IU per day, depending on your general lifestyle. People who don't exercise, who smoke, and who consume high amounts of alcoholic beverages will need the higher dosage. Those with a more moderate lifestyle can get by with lower levels of supplementation.

Food sources of Vitamin E

Wheat germ oil: 32.2 IU per 1 Tb

Sunflower seeds: 26.8 IU per ¼ cup

Almonds: 12.7 IU per ¼ cup

Sweet potato: 9 IU per medium potato

Tempeh: 8.5 IU per 2oz

Flax oil: 7.5 IU per 1Tb

Buckwheat flour: 5.8 IU per ½ cup

Vitamin B6

Vitamin B6 is an important vitamin for mucous membrane integrity, which is your immune system's first line of defense against invaders. B6 is needed to produce B

and T-lymphocytic cells. B6 is also involved in the
formation of body proteins, neurotransmitters, maintaining
hormone balance and in red blood cell production. Current
recommendations for B6 supplementation range from
1.7mcg-40 mcg a day. Signs of B6 deficiency are
depression, glucose intolerance and impaired nerve
function.[13] Zinc is required as a cofactor to activate vitamin
B6 for mucous membrane integrity.

Food Sources of B6 (per 3 ½ oz. serving)

Brewer's yeast: 3 mg

Sunflower seeds: 1.25 mg

Walnuts: 0.73 mg

Brown rice: 0.55 mg

Bananas: 0.51 mg

Avocado: 0.42 mg

Bioflavonoids

Bioflavonoids make up the color components of plants.
Over 4000 different flavonoid compounds have been
identified. In humans, bioflavonoids act as biological
response modifiers. They are able to modify the body's
response to allergens, viruses, and cancer causing agents.
Bioflavonoids demonstrate anti-inflammatory, anti-viral,
anti-allergic, and anti-cancer activities in many studies.

They have a supportive effect on collagen, reinforcing
natural cross-linkage. Collagen integrity helps keep tissues
healthy and supports the body's first line of defense against

germs. They enhance the action of vitamin C and prevent damage to muscles and organs by acting as an anti-oxidant. Bioflavonoids are most concentrated in green vegetables and some fruit.

Food Sources of Bioflavonoids

Blueberries, black currants, black raspberries, cherries, cranberries, hawthorn berries, oranges, tomatoes, onions, sage, green tea, red wine, red grapes, chocolate.

Minerals for Immune Health

Selenium

Selenium increases natural killer cells and mobilizes cancer-fighting cells. It is also a component of an antioxidant system that works with vitamin E to prevent cellular damage. Low levels of selenium are associated with cancer, cardiovascular disease, inflammatory conditions, and premature aging.[14]

Recommended daily intake is 200 mcg a day. Over 2000 mcg a day produces toxicity.

Food Sources of Selenium (per 3 ½ oz.)

Wheat germ: 111 mcg

Brazil nuts: 103 mcg

Barley/ Whole wheat bread: 66 mcg

Bran: 63 mcg

Red swiss chard: 57 mcg

Turnips: 27 mcg

Garlic: 25 mcg

Zinc

This valuable mineral increases your body's production of white blood cells (the infection fighters) and helps them fight more aggressively by releasing more antibodies. It also increases cancer-fighting natural killer cells. Zinc is required as a cofactor to activate vitamin B6 for mucous membrane integrity.

Zinc increases the number of infection-fighting T-cells, especially in elderly people who are often deficient in zinc and whose immune systems often weaken with age.

For infants and children, there is some evidence dietary zinc supplements may reduce the incidence of acute respiratory infections and may decrease the duration of acute diarrhea. The best sources of zinc for infants and young children are foods high in zinc and zinc-fortified cereals.

Zinc in excess of 75 milligrams a day can inhibit immune function.[15] You can ask your physician to check your zinc status. A zinc WBC levels is the best indicator for zinc status and a zinc tally test also can detect low zinc status.[16]

Food sources of Zinc

Oysters, eastern: 113 mg per ½ cup

Beef, roast: 5.3 mg per 3 oz.

Cheese, cheddar and swiss: 3.3 mg per 3oz.

Swiss chard: 3.2 mg per 1 cup.

Oats, rolled: 2.8 mg per 1 cup.

Pumpkin seeds: 2.6 mg per ¼ cup

Garlic and the Immune System

Garlic is a powerful immune booster. It stimulates the production of infection-fighting white blood cells, boosts natural killer cell activity, and increases the efficiency of natural antibody production. The immune-boosting properties of garlic seem to be due to its sulfur-containing compounds, such as allicin and sulfides.[17]

Garlic can also act as an antioxidant by reducing the build-up of free radicals in the bloodstream. Garlic has anti-platelet activity, promoting cardiovascular health. Garlic may also protect against many different cancers, helps the liver detoxify, lowers cholesterol, helps to normalize blood sugar in Type 2 Diabetes, and reduces high blood pressure.

Eating raw garlic and/or cooking with garlic are the best ways to consume it.   However, if you, or more importantly, others around you, do not appreciate the smell of garlic de-odorized garlic in capsule form is also effective. Eating a few sprigs of parsley can also reduce the aroma of garlic on the breath. Three cloves of garlic a day is recommended when you are sick and three cloves of garlic a week for preventative measures.[18]

Healthy Oils and the Immune System

Essential Fatty Acids

There are two kinds of essential fatty acids: omega-3 and omega-6. Fatty acids are needed for hormones and neurotransmitter production, they decrease platelet aggregation, support the immune system, are anti-inflammatory, promote skin/membrane health, normalize cholesterol and utilization of the Vitamins A, D, E, K. Without essential fatty acids, the body holds on to excess fat.[19]

The omega-3 fatty acids in flax oil and fatty fish (such as salmon, tuna, and mackerel) act as immune boosters by increasing the activity of phagocytes (the bacteria-eating white blood cells). Cod liver oil, not flax oil, also contains vitamin A which adds additional immune support.

Essential fatty acids also protect the body against damage from over-reactions to infection. When you take essential fatty acid supplements, such as flax or fish oils, take additional vitamin E, usually 400 IU a day, which acts together with essential fatty acids to boost the immune system.

Children taking a half teaspoon of flax oil a day experienced fewer and less severe respiratory infections and fewer school absences, in a recent study.

Possible Signs of Essential Fatty Acid Deficiency
- Hyperkeratosis: Small hard bumps on cheeks, outside surface of upper arms and/or thighs
- Impacted earwax in ears
- Dry rough skin, dry brittle hair
- Diet high in animal fats with little to no fish

Food Sources of Essential Fatty Acids
- *Omega-3 sources*: salmon, cod, mackerel, halibut, flax seed, hemp, canola, walnut, pumpkin, and soy oil
- *Omega-6 sources*: nuts, seeds, grains, safflower, sunflower, soy, sesame, corn, olive oil, and cottonseed

Both omega-3 and omega-6 fatty acids should be refrigerated and not heated at any point. Heating changes the oils into trans-fats that are detrimental to your cell membranes. Cooking fish will not drastically change the omega oils in fish.

Increasing Fatty Acids in Diet

- Add 1-3 teaspoons flax or cod liver oil to a fruit and yogurt smoothie
- Use flax oil in salad dressings
- Pour flax oil over salads, grains, or veggies
- Eat more wild, cold, deep water fish such as salmon, halibut, mackerel, herring, sardines, etc.
- Switch to using certain vegetable oils such as canola oil, flaxseed oil, and walnut oil alone or mixed with olive oil.

Medium Chain Fatty Acids

Medium chain fatty acids (MCFA) are a type of fatty acid found in coconut oil, palm kernel oil, milk fat and butter. MCFA demonstrate anti-bacterial, anti-viral action in multiple studies.[20] MCFA will spilt open the membrane of the organism by disrupting their lipid membrane. MCFA kill invading organisms without causing any known harm to human tissues. Different types of MCFA have various antimicrobial actions. For example caprylic acid and capric acid are antimicrobial while lauric acid provides the most anti-viral action.[21] Coconut oil contains 48% lauric acid, 7% capric acid, and 8% caprylic acid. Palm kernel oil also contains up to 50% lauric acid. Butter and milk fat contain about 3%. Adding 1-3 Tb of coconut oil is a promising way to destroy many bacteria and viruses.

Better Butter[22]

Soften butter by sitting it out on the counter for several hours. Mix butter and flaxseed, olive oil, or coconut oil in a 1:1 ratio. Place in a closed container in the refrigerator to harden again. Adding flax or olive oil softens the butter, adds a delicious flavor and supplies cholesterol-lowering essential fatty acids to the saturated butterfat. Coconut oil supplies anti-bacterial lauric acid.

Nutrition During Illness

Most people, especially children, don't feel like eating during or following a cold or illness. Consequently, their nutrition suffers and their immune system suffers. This cycle accounts for the common occurrence of getting one infection after another. It's best to keep your body well nourished, so it has nutritional reserves to withstand several days of poor eating.

Eating or drinking something like the *Immune Support Smoothie* or the *Immune Support Breakfast* daily for two weeks during times of increased exposure (as listed below) can support your immune system.

- beginning of the school year
- beginning daycare
- coworker, family member or friend is sick
- you or your child feel a cold coming on
- travel on an airplane, cruise, bus or
- around a large number of people

Nutrition Tips for Children

How Can I Get My Child to Eat Healthy Foods?

Getting your child involved, experimenting with food presentation, and hiding vegetables in different food preparations are all ways to increase your child's intake of healthy foods.

Involving your child in buying food, food preparation, serving meals, and cleaning up are all ways of creating a healthy relationship with food.[23] For older children, planting a garden or going to a farm to harvest vegetables familiarizes children with the source of fruits and vegetables, making them more interesting.

Food preparation is a big deal for children. Decorating food, using special plates and cups and telling a story about individual dishes are all great ways to make eating different foods more exciting.

Examples of Ways to Make Food Interesting[24]:

- Use a cookie cutter of your child's favorite animal or other shapes to cut carrots, whole-grain pancakes, and sandwiches
- Use an ice cream scoop to serve brown rice or mashed potatoes as miniature mountains
- Make a face on food with raisins, small vegetables, crackers (use your imagination)

- Make up a story about melted gold when serving yellow split pea soup or make a plate of spaghetti into pretend hay for sheep, horses, or elephants
- Tell a story so incredible your child can't resist tasting the dish

Disguising vegetables in many different dishes is another great way to increase vegetable consumption:

- Add carrot or beet juice to apple juice and dilute it in half with water (this cuts down on sugar while increasing vegetables in the diet)
- Add vegetables to a soup and then puree the soup to disguise the vegetables
- Add vegetables to muffins or other baked goods
- Mix vegetables in sandwich spreads
- Mix grated carrots, zucchini, corn or green peppers to a burrito or other foods (see *Ham Fried Rice* recipe).[25]

Optimal Digestion

It's not enough just to purchase and serve organic whole foods. Proper digestion plays a major role in our body's absorbing all the nutrients. Here are some general guidelines for improving digestion:

Mindful Eating

- Relax before eating. Allow 30 seconds of deep breathing and/or affirmation about digestion, nourishment and for saying "grace".[1] Be grateful for what you eat. Let food be a ritual of celebration and joy.

- Notice *why* you are eating.
- Eat sitting down in a relaxed place. When you eat—just eat. No studying, worrying, or arguing. Eating is a self-nourishing act; allow time for this.

Eat Slowly

- Chew foods thoroughly and eat slowly to set the stage for proper digestive enzyme release. The pancreas only releases enzymes when it receives sufficient salivary and gastric stimulation.
- Avoid drinking beverages during a meal or 20 minutes before or after. Drinking dilutes the stomach acid needed to break down proteins and absorb minerals. If you are thirsty during a meal, you probably aren't chewing well enough (or you haven't been drinking water throughout the day). Chewing should create enough saliva and moistness.
- If you are in a rush, eating a small meal in a relaxed fashion is more beneficial than eating a large meal quickly. You will actually absorb more nutrients from the small meal.[ii]

Regular meals

- Eat meals around the same time each day. This trains the body to release and produce enzymes at appropriate times.
- No food should be eaten 2 hours before bedtime.

Digestive Aids

Sometimes the body needs assistance digesting foods. Digestive aids taken 10 minutes before a meal (such as herbal bitters, apple cider vinegar, or lemon juice) stimulate your stomach and prepare it to digest. Usually one teaspoon is needed to stimulate digestion.

Some people need more support to maintain optimal digestion and absorption of nutrients. Betaine HCL and pancreatic enzymes supplement your body's natural stomach acid and pancreatic enzymes respectively. Digestive enzymes are often needed by those who have a history of poor eating habits: eating quickly, poor quality food, eating on the go, erratic eating habits (not eating at the same time every day).

You may also need digestive enzymes if you are under a great deal of stress. When your body is under stress (physical, mental, or social), your nervous system shunts blood to the muscles and brain. This is called the "fight or flight" response. For optimal digestion, you need the opposite response: "rest and digest." If you eat during the "fight or flight" response, you will have less stomach acid and pancreatic enzymes to digest the food and less blood going to the digestive tract to absorb nutrients.

Over time, a pattern of eating under stress creates protein and mineral deficiencies directly affecting your immune and hormone system. To reverse this cycle, follow the mindful eating guidelines discussed previously and take digestive enzymes to rebuild your digestive system function.

Do I Need Digestive Support?

You may need digestive support if you experience:

- nausea after eating
- a feeling of fullness or heaviness in the stomach that lasts over two hours
- bloating, gas, constipation, or diarrhea
- fatigue or exhaustion after eating
- bad breath

---

[1] Murray, MT. (1993). *The healing power of foods.* Rocklin, CA: Prima Publishing.

[2] Lair, C. (1997). Feeding the whole family: Whole foods recipes for babies, young children and their parents. Moon Smile Press: Seattle, WA.

[3] National Organic Program. Background Information retrieved May 12, 2006 from
http://www.ams.usda.gov/nop/FactSheets/Backgrounder.html

[4] Lu C, et al. (2006). Organic diets significantly lower children's dietary exposure to organophosphorus pesticides. Environmental Health Perspectives. 114: 260-263.

[5] Lehey, Stephen. (2006) New studies back benefit of organic diet. *Interpress Services* retrieved May 11, 2006 from
http://www.organicconsumers.org/2006/article_91.cfm

[6] Zahm SH, Ward MH.(1998). Pesticides and childhood cancer. *Environmental Health Perspectives*, 106 Suppl 3:893-908.

[7] Daniels JL, Olshan AF, Savitz DA.(1997). Pesticides and childhood cancers. *Environmental Health Perspectives*, 105:1068-77.

[8] Zahm SII.(1999). Childhood leukemia and pesticides (commentary). *Epidemiology*, 10:473-475.

[9] Infante-Rivard C, Labuda D, Krajinovic M, Sinnett D. (1999). Risk of childhood leukemia associated with exposure to pesticides and with gene polymorphisms. *Epidemiology*, 10:481-7.

[10] Retrieved 11/22/2016 from https://www.ewg.org/foodnews/dirty_dozen_list.php EWG's 2016 Shopper's Guide to Pesticides in Produce™

[11] Bove, Mary. (2001). *An encyclopedia of natural healing for children and infants.* Chicago, IL Keats.

[12] Aranow, C. (2011). Vitamin D and the Immune System. *Journal of Investigative Medicine : The Official Publication of the American Federation for Clinical Research*, 59(6), 881–886. http://doi.org/10.231/JIM.0b013e31821b8755

[13] Murray, MT. (1993). *The healing power of foods.* Rocklin, CA: Prima Publishing.

[14] Murray, MT. (1993). *The healing power of foods.* Rocklin, CA: Prima Publishing.

[15] Marz, RB. (1999). *Medical Nutrition from Marz* (2nd ed.). Portland, OR: Omni-Press.

[16] Marz, RB. (1999). *Medical Nutrition from Marz* (2nd ed.). Portland, OR: Omni-Press.

[17] Colic, M and Savic, M. (2000). Garlic extracts stimulate proliferation of rat lymphocytes in vitro by increasing IL-2 and IL-4 production. *Immunopharmacology and Immunotoxicology.* Feb;22(1):163-81.

[18] Murray, MT. (1993). *The healing power of foods.* Rocklin, CA: Prima Publishing.

[19] Marz, RB. (1999). *Medical Nutrition from Marz* (2nd ed.). Portland, OR: Omni-Press.

[20] Fife, Bruce. (2004). *The coconut oil miracle.* New York: Avery.

[21] Fife, Bruce. (2004). *The coconut oil miracle.* New York: Avery.

[22] Balch, Phyllis and James. (2000). *Prescriptions for Nutritional Healing,* (3rd ed.). New York: Avery.

[23] Lair, C. (1997). *Feeding the whole family: Whole foods recipes for babies, young children and their parents.* Seattle: Moon Smile Press.

[24] Lair, C. (1997). *Feeding the whole family: Whole foods recipes for babies, young children and their parents.* Seattle: Moon Smile Press.

[25] Lair, C. (1997). *Feeding the whole family: Whole foods recipes for babies, young children and their parents.* Seattle: Moon Smile Press.

6 | Immune Botanicals

For centuries, our ancestors used herbs to improve health and treat disease. Many used herbs traditionally to treat infection, inflammation, and to strengthen the immune system. Herbs beneficial to the immune system can be classified into two main categories:

Supportive herbs (Immunomodulators) work by decreasing the effects of stress on your body while supporting your adrenal glands and your immune system. This combination of support and protection against stress balances the immune system response. Supportive herbs are traditionally taken for long periods of time to tonify and strengthen the immune and nervous systems.

Stimulating herbs act by stimulating different parts of the immune system. Because of their stimulating effect, they should only be taken for a short period of time and then discontinued for a week or two. Taking stimulating herbs for an extended period of time can "wear out" your immune system and leave you prone to frequent colds and bouts of flu.

Most immune stimulating herbs and some immune supportive herbs are contraindicated in pregnancy. Always check with your naturopathic physician or health care provider skilled in herbal medicine before taking any herbs while pregnant or nursing.

Immune Supportive Herbs

Immunomodulating herbs act by normalizing the immune system's response. This means if the immune system is deficient, immunomodulating herbs strengthen it; if the immune system is overactive (as in autoimmune conditions such as Rheumatoid arthritis and Lupus) immunomodulating herbs normalize the immune system response.

Immunomodulators are excellent in helping to normalize immune responses in allergic asthma, hay fever, food allergies, hives, and interstitial cystitis. They should also be a major part of any preventative strategy, especially if there is a history of frequent colds, flu's or infections. By taking immune supportive herbs, you can strengthen and balance your immune system response without overstimulation.

All of the herbs listed below are immunomodulating herbs. (For help with herbal terms, see the *Glossary*.)

American Ginseng (*Panax quinquifolius*): Increases resistance to stress, increases mental alertness, enhances natural killer cells, raises all neurotransmitter levels except serotonin, and normalizes blood sugar. American ginseng is less stimulating than Asian ginseng. It is indicated for excessive dry cough and dry mouth.

Asian Ginseng (*Panax ginseng)*: Most studied of all adaptogens. Especially indicated for weakness, fatigue, low body temperature, insomnia related to extreme depletion, and stress-related immune suppression. Asian ginseng can be very stimulating. It's a powerful herb to aid in rejuvenation and increasing vitality in the elderly or chronically ill. If Asian ginseng is too stimulating, switch to American ginseng.

Ashwagandha (*Withania somnifera*): anti-inflammatory, decreases blood pressure, modulates all kinds of stressors, prevents stress-induced ulcers, increases thyroid hormone conversion to a more active form, and is anti-bacterial. Overall it promotes physical and mental health and arrests the aging process. It alleviates depression and anxiety.

Astragalus (*Astragalus membranaceus*): good tonic for the immune system, builds and strengthens the entire body, improves digestion and assimilation of nutrients. Best tonic for those under 35 years. Studies have shown after a few months use, an increase in antibody levels and increased lymphocytes. It is also useful in supporting patients undergoing chemotherapy and radiation (to increase red and white blood cell counts) when taken in much higher doses than usual.

Holy Basil (*Ocimum sanctum*): anti-inflammatory, immune supporting, inhibits allergic asthma, improves cognitive function, and stabilizes blood sugar.

Licorice root (*Glycyrrhiza glabra*): estrogenic, immune supporting, modulates stress response, aids in expectoration, anti-viral, and soothes sore throats. Licorice root may exacerbate high blood pressure and should be avoided if this occurs.

Reishi/Ganoderma Mushrooms *(Ganoderma)*: powerful immunomodulator especially in patients with difficulty sleeping, fatigue, poor memory, allergic asthma, and autoimmune conditions.

Asian mushrooms such as Reishi and Maitake are deep immune tonics often used in cancer treatment and in stress related immune suppression. They stimulate all parts of the immune system while lowering cholesterol and triglycerides. Countless studies over the last 40 years have confirmed the ability of these mushrooms to stimulate a variety of immune components.

Schisandra fruit *(Schisandra chinensis)*: provides strong immune support for the kidneys, lungs and upper respiratory tract, stabilizes mast cells and reduces histamine response to reduce allergy symptoms in asthma and hay fever.

Siberian Ginseng (*Eleutherococcus senticosus*): especially indicated for low vitality and endurance due to stress. Specifically increases lymphocyte activity (anti-viral). Very useful in chronic disease states to increase immune activity and for adrenal support.

Immune Stimulating Herbs

Immune stimulating herbs should not be used for longer than a two week period before having a break for a week or two. Immune stimulating herbs should not be used if you have an autoimmune condition. If you are pregnant or nursing, seek the advice of a Naturopathic physician or doctor skilled in herbal medicine.

Echinacea (*Echinacea angustifolia*): anti-viral, immune stimulating, and anti-bacterial by preventing the spread of bacteria through tissue. Best used when one is physically run down due to work or physical exercise.

Grapefruit Seed Extract: anti-viral, anti-bacterial, and anti-fungal action especially indicated for candida and parasite infections.

Lomatium *(Lomatium dissectum)*: comparable to penicillin in anti-bacterial action, great for chronic fatigue due to viral infections and upper respiratory tract infections.

Osha *(Ligusticum porteri)*: especially indicated for upper respiratory tract infections (at the beginning of the infection) and nagging coughs (at the end of the infection).

Usnea (*Old Man's Beard*): better than penicillin, great for trichomonas infection and most other infections.

Essential oils are anti-bacterial, anti-viral and anti-fungal when used on the skin or in a steam tent. Combination formulas such as Thieves oil are formulated to stimulate the immune system and kill germs. Essential oils should not be used internally, unless under the care of a Naturopathic physician.

Anti-Bacterial Herbs

Chaparral *(Larrea tridentata)*: kills and prevents infection and is anti-inflammatory.

Goldenseal *(Hydrastis canadensis)*: wonderful anti-bacterial for any mucous membrane infection: urinary tract infection, upper respiratory tract infection, sinus infection.

Spilanthes *(Spilanthes)*: best for mouth or throat infections, immune stimulating, works well with echinacea. Increases appetite in sickness.

Anti-Viral Herbs

Calendula *(Calendula officinalis)*: anti-viral for the lower body, immune stimulating, and anti-inflammatory. Calendula stimulates white blood cell activity and lymphatic activity to help clear an infection, as in chronic respiratory infections. Calendula will help heal the digestive tract after diarrhea or food poisoning and lifts the spirits in seasonal affective disorder.

Pokeroot (*Phytolacca*): anti-viral, lymph stimulant for hard nodes (specifically for head, neck and breast infections/inflammations). Best to use in small doses combined with other herbs as it can be toxic in large doses.

Oil of Oregano: anti-viral and anti-fungal activity, calms the stomach, decreases coughing, especially good for sore throats and treating fungal infections.

St. John's Wort (*Hypericum perforatum*): St. John's Wort has gained notoriety for its mood enhancing effects, but is also anti-viral and useful in chronic viral conditions, stomach viruses and respiratory viruses. St. John's Wort also calms irritability and decreases nerve related pain. Some people have experienced a rash when taking St John's Wort and then being exposed to sunlight. Discontinue use if this occurs.

Immune Support/Stimulation for Children

For centuries, parents have used herbs to treat childhood colds, flus, and bacterial infections. The herbs most commonly used for children are immune stimulating in a gentle way and have many other synergistic effects. For example, chamomile is antimicrobial and antiseptic but also decreases nausea, intestinal gas, and irritability. These herbs usually taste better than some given to adults and all have been proven safe for children.

Immune Supportive Herbs for Children

Astragalus (*Astragalus membranaceus*): Astragalus is the best immune supportive herb for children and young adults. It is a wonderful tonic that stimulates white blood cell production and natural killer cells. It is most helpful in building up the immune system in chronic disease, allergies, and reoccurring infections. It is often combined with nettles, licorice, and calendula flowers to build up the immune system in children.

Ashwagandha (*Withania somnifera*) Ashwagandha is an adaptogen, immunomodulator, tonic, anti-inflammatory, and a mild sedative. This herb is most indicated for calming the body and emotions while increasing stress-coping action (especially after physical trauma or severe illness). It promotes growth in young children and is indicated for children who experience weight loss and failure to grow (common signs of stress in children).

Siberian Ginseng *(Eleutherococcus senticosus)*: Siberian Ginseng is an adaptogen, immunomodulatory, and tonic. Siberian ginseng is best used to strengthen the immune system after antibiotic use, a high fever, prolonged illness, surgery, or for children who get sick after stressful situations. It increases concentration, memory, and returns vitality to a weakened system.

Immune Stimulating Herbs for Children

Chamomile *(Chamomile spp.)*: Chamomile is an excellent herb for most colds and infections. Chamomile is antimicrobial, antiseptic, carminative, relaxant, and decreases diarrhea, nausea, and vomiting. Chamomile helps break up and move out excessive mucus in the sinuses and upper airways.

Cinnamon: Cinnamon is antimicrobial, carminative, kills intestinal worms and increases circulation. Cinnamon is especially indicated in influenza infections and for intestinal worms. It can be mixed with carob powder and applesauce to stop diarrhea and added to teas with other immune stimulating herbs.

Echinacea *(Echinacea angustifolia or purpurea)*: Echinacea is anti-viral, immune stimulant (by stimulating nonspecific immune response), increases white blood cells and lymphocyte activity at the site of infection and increases macrophage ability to eat bacteria, fungus, and viruses. The fresh juice is anti-viral against herpes and influenza viruses. Works well as a throat gargle for tonsillitis, laryngitis, and mouth ulcers.

Elder flowers and berries *(Sambucus nigra)*: Elder stimulates nonspecific immune function, is diaphoretic and anticatarrhal. The berries are anti-viral, anti-inflammatory, and immune tonics. The flowers stimulate nonspecific immune function especially in the upper airways and sinuses. Elder flowers encourage sweating to bring down a high fever.

Hyssop *(Hyssopus officinalis)*: Hyssop is anti-bacterial, antifungal, antispasmodic, and helps expectorate mucous. It is indicated for dry coughs such as whooping cough. It is a good antiseptic throat gargle.

Lemon balm *(Melissa officinalis)*: Lemon balm is antiviral, circulatory stimulant, diaphoretic, antidepressant, and carminative. It is best used as an essential oil in a steam tent for antimicrobial action on the respiratory passages and to elevate mood. The tea helps to calm an upset stomach.

Licorice root *(Glycerrhiza glabra)*: Licorice is antiviral, anti-inflammatory, and an expectorant. It stimulates natural killer cells and macrophages to inhibit viral activity. Licorice is very helpful for any childhood viral disease: chickenpox, herpes, measles, or any viral infection. It soothes dry spastic coughs and soothes sore throats.

Peppermint *(Mentha piperita)*: Peppermint is antiseptic, relieves digestive upset, gas, and nausea. Spearmint also has the same properties, but is more mild and easier to give to children.

Sage *(Salvia officinalis)*: Sage is antimicrobial and antiseptic specifically for the throat and mouth. Sage will dry up mucus secretions and works well as a gargle to treat sore throats by reducing irritation and acting as an antiseptic.

St. John's Wort *(Hypericum perforatum)*: See adult description.

Thyme *(Thymus vulgaris)*: Thyme is one of the best herbs for respiratory tract infections such as bronchitis and pneumonia. Thyme is anti-bacterial and anti-viral and is useful for all types of coughs. It breaks up congestion, warms the mucous membranes and helps the body expel mucus. It is best in decreasing spastic dry coughs. Thyme also calms the stomach and digestive tract and soothes sore throats.

Herbs for Symptom Relief in Adults and Children

Catnip *(Nepeta cateria)*: Catnip is carminative, diaphoretic, relaxant, and mild sedative. Catnip is most indicated to help soothe stomach and intestinal pain, calm or quiet an irritable child and for children with high fevers (over 101.5) by promoting sweating. Often combined with yarrow and elder flower as a tea or in a bath to comfort, soothe, and decrease a fever.

Elecampane *(Inula helenium)*: Elecampane is antitussive, bitter, and expectorant. Elecampane is most indicated in a dry nonproductive (not much mucus) cough by thinning mucus and aiding in expectorating. It also decreases spasms in the chest often seen in bronchitis, asthma, and bronchial pneumonia.

Slippery Elm *(Ulmus rubra)*: Slippery elm is most indicated in a burning, hot tummy, diarrhea, nausea, and vomiting. Slippery Elm throat lozenges are available to soothe sore throats. It is most often used as a powder and added to oatmeal or applesauce.

Yarrow (*Achillea millefolium*): Yarrow is an anti-inflammatory, diaphoretic, and carminative. This combination makes yarrow very effective to treat colds and flus with swollen glands, decreased appetite, stomach and intestinal pain, and a high fever. Yarrow is most often combined with elder flower and peppermint and taken as a tea to treat the above conditions.

Immune Stimulating Herbs by Body System

Digestive System

> Calendula *(Calendula officinalis)*
> Chamomile (*Chamomile spp.*)
> Echinacea (*Echinacea angustifolia*)
> Myrrh (*Commiphora molmol*)
> Thyme (*Thymus vulgaris*)
> Wormwood (*Artemisia absinthum*)

Kidney

> Bearberry (*Arctostaphylos uva-ursi)*
> Buchu (*Barosma betulina*)
> Garlic (*Allium sativum*)
> Juniper (*Juniperus communis*)

Respiratory System

Anise *(Pimpinella anisum)*
Echinacea *(Echinacea angustifolia)*
Garlic *(Allium sativum)*
Goldenseal *(Hydrastis canadensis)*
Lomatium *(Lomatium dissectum)*
Osha *(Ligusticum porteri)*
Pleurisy root *(Asclepias tuberosa)*
Thyme *(Thymus vulgaris)*
Wild Indigo *(Baptisia tinctoria)*

Skin

Calendula *(Calendula officinalis)*
Chickweed *(Stellaria media)*
Echinacea *(Echinacea angustifolia)*
Goldenseal *(Hydrastis canadensis)*
Myrrh *(Commiphora molmol)*
Wild Indigo *(Baptisia tinctoria)*

How Much Should I Take?

The doses suggested below are general recommendations. Please read the instructions on any supplement or tincture you buy and take the recommended dose, unless directed to do otherwise by your natural health care provider.

For acute conditions (3-5 days) take:
> Tea: 1 Tb/cup, drink 5-8 cups a day
> Tincture: 1 tsp, every two-three hours (6-8 times a day)
> Capsules: 2 capsules, every 3 hours
> Syrup: 1 Tb, 3-6 times a day
> Herbal milk: 1 tsp powdered herb/1 cup milk, three times a day

For long term support (3 weeks or more) take:
> Tea: 1Tb/cup, drink 3 cups a day
> Tincture: 1 tsp, 2-3 times a day
> Capsules: 3 capsules, 2 times a day
> Syrup: 1 Tb, 2-3 times a day.
> Herbal milk: 1 tsp powdered herb/1 cup milk, once a day

Dosing for Children

Most herbal formulas for children display the appropriate dose on the bottle. If you are using an adult product, you will need to adjust the dose accordingly. Always consult your naturopathic physician or pediatrician if any condition continues for more than a few days or if there is a high fever.

Clark's Rule

> Child's weight in pounds/150 lb. = fraction of adult dose
> Example: 50 lb. child/150 lb. = 1/3 adult dose

General Dosing for Children by Weight

Weight of Child	Tea	Tincture
Doses per day	Acute: 5-8 times Chronic: 3 times	Acute: 6-8 times Chronic: 2-3 times
5-15 lb.	2 tablespoons	2-3 drops
16-35 lb.	¼ cup	¼ tsp
36-65 lb.	½ cup	½ tsp
66-80 lb.	¾ cup	¾ tsp
81-110 lb. Adult dose	1 cup	1 tsp

How Can I Get My Child To Take Herbal Medicine?

The secret in getting children to take herbal medicine is to hide the flavor in something that tastes good, such as juice, honey (not for infants less than 1 year) homemade popsicles, syrup, or a glycerite tincture. Adding a regular tincture to juice the child can drink or freezing the juice mixture into popsicles provides a great way to get kids to take herbs.

Herbal popsicles and syrups are high in sugar (which suppresses the immune system), but the benefit of taking the herbs in an acute setting (2-3 days) outweighs this suppression.

You can also add immune herbs to foods, such as adding astragalus root to soups or adding tinctures to applesauce or other foods to hide the flavor.

Herbal Syrups

Syrups are most indicated for respiratory conditions such as coughs or irritated sore throats. Syrup is made by combining a tincture, infusion, or decoction with sugar, honey, or glycerine. Herbs that combine well in a syrup are licorice, ginger, garlic, elder, lemon balm, cinnamon, fennel, and cayenne. Syrups can last one month if refrigerated. (See the recipe section for a few ideas).

Glycerite tincture

A glycerite tincture is made from glycerine: a sweet substance that preserves and extracts the key parts of the herb. Glycerites are a great way for kids to take herbs regularly as the sweetness hides some of the herbal taste.

Herbal Popsicles

Herbal popsicles can be made by combining tincture, infusions, or decoctions with juice and then freezing the mixture. Usually it takes 2 hours to freeze. Herbal popsicles soothe hot irritated sore throats and provide a way for kids to take herbs.

Herbal paste

Herbal pastes can be made with powdered herbs mixed with honey until a thick consistency is created. Herbs that work well in pastes are cinnamon, licorice, ginger, fennel, and chamomile. Give herbal pastes in ¼ to ½ tsp doses two or more times a day.

Herb-infused bath

You can also add tea to a bath and have your child soak for at least a half hour. Herb infused baths are a great way for little ones to absorb the herbs and their healing aromatic oils. This works extremely well with aromatic herbs which smell good, such as elder, chamomile, and yarrow. The herb-infused bath also provides steam inhalation to break up mucus in the upper airways and relax your child to promote sleeping and decrease aches and pains associated with getting a cold or flu.

To make an herb-infused bath, make two quarts of tea by steeping 2 cups of herbs in two quarts of tea for 20 minutes and add it to a bath.

Another quick way to make an herbal bath is to put two cups of herbs into a tube sock or cotton bag and attach it to the spout of the tub. Run the water through the herbs and then tie off the sock or cotton bag and have it float in the bath. It is not as strong as making a tea first, but it is more convenient.

Essential oils such as lavender, thyme, and calendula can also be added to provide additional anti-bacterial, anti-viral and calming action. (Usually about 5 drops each) Elder flowers, yarrow, and catnip combine well to decrease a high fever (over 101.5), decrease aches, and pains and calm the body.[1]

If your child is extremely achy, adding 1 cup of Epsom salts to the bath provides magnesium that can relax tight muscles from coughing or just the aches of a cold or flu.

---

[1] Bove, Mary.(2001). An encyclopedia of natural healing for children and infants. Keats: Chicago, IL.

7 | **When You Are Sick**

What to do when you begin to feel sick

At the first sign of cold/flu: i.e. sore throat, fatigue:

- Take Oscillococcinum: 10 pellets every few hours
- Take Ferrum phos30c: 3 pellets every few hours
- Do the *Warming Sock* or *Warming Body* hydrotherapy treatment
- Take immune-stimulating/anti-bacterial/anti-viral herbs
- Get plenty of sleep, eat nutrient dense foods, NO SUGAR!
- Enjoy specific topical treatments (mustard pack, nasal irrigation, carrot poultice, or homemade vapor rub)
- Pinpoint why you got sick and change immunosuppressive behaviors

Plan Your Attack

To be victorious in your battle against germ invaders, be specific in your attack strategy. Determine whether your symptoms match a bacterial, viral, or influenza infection. You can then direct your attack appropriately by choosing herbs best for fighting bacteria or viruses.

An additional strategy is to classify your body's reaction to the infection-- either hot or cold. Once you know the type of infection and your body's reaction, you can select specific herbs to more efficiently fight off the infection.

Symptoms over the course of an illness often change. There may be the initial reaction of fever, chills, aches, fatigue, and/or sore throat which changes to more of the clean-up stage with coughing, lots of mucus (dead white blood cells and invaders) and overall congestion from the your body's battle against the invader. Changing the herbs you use according to the stage of your illness can really speed up your recovery time and decrease your symptoms.

Herbs are powerful allies in the fight against infection. Studies with American ginseng showed the rate of developing two or more colds during a 4-month period was 50% less in the ginseng group than in the placebo group. The total number of cold symptom days were 5-6 days shorter for the ginseng group than the placebo group.[1]

Virus vs. Bacteria

Bacterial infections usually have these symptoms:

- persistently high fever
- thick, colored nasal discharge
- chronic cough
- last longer than 2 weeks

Viral infections usually have these symptoms:

- runny nose
- watery eyes
- dry cough
- sore throat
- chills, aches, and pains
- mild or no fever
- lasts about 7 days

If in doubt about your infection, consult your naturopathic physician and take herbs that are anti-viral/anti-bacterial and immune stimulating.

Is it a Cold or the Flu?

Colds generally require minimal-moderate immune and anti-viral support where flu symptoms can be debilitating and last for weeks. If you have the flu, you should hit it hard with immune stimulating and anti-viral herbs while eliminating immune suppressing activity.

Flu symptoms include a high fever (100-102°F) for 2-3 days (different from most viral infections that have mild or no fever), headache, general aches and pains that are severe, fatigue and weakness for 2-3 weeks, extreme exhaustion, cough that worsens, sneezing, and stuffy nose. Your MD may want to prescribe anti-viral medications if the symptoms are severe or persistent.

Cold symptoms include slight aches and pains, mild fatigue, stuffy nose, sneezing, coughing, and sore throat.

Hot vs. Cold Reaction

If you classify your symptoms as either hot or cold, you can increase your success at fighting off invaders quickly by balancing your body's response. Every herb has an ability to warm the body, cool the body, or be neutral. Balancing your body's response to an illness can help tremendously in recovering quickly and symptom improvement. Neutral herbs good for both conditions are slippery elm, licorice, and chamomile.

Hot reactions to infections usually produce symptoms like having a red face, being loud and talkative, an irritable attitude, sweating easily, a high fever with slight chills, thirsty, dry mouth, strong appetite, preference for cooling foods and drinks.[2]

If there you have a hot reaction, choose immune herbs to cool the system. Cooling herbs include echinacea, elder flower, lemon balm, mullein, and plantain.

Cold reactions to infections usually produce symptoms such as a pale face, being tired and quiet, sleeping a lot, cold skin temperature and feet feeling cold, low fever but strong chills, no thirst, poor appetite, loose stools or diarrhea, and preference for warm food or drinks.[3]

If you have a cold reaction, choose immune herbs to warm the system. Warming herbs include cayenne, cinnamon, ginger, calendula, yarrow, garlic, and fennel.

How Do I Know Which Herbs to Pick?

Choosing from the vast amount of herbs available can be quite daunting. The easiest way to start is to pick herbs with immune stimulating, anti-bacterial, and anti-viral properties. Other ways to pick herbs are[4]:

- Choose herbs easy to find or available
- Choose herbs according to the hot or cold reaction of your body
- Choose herbs to match your specific symptoms

Allow the Immune System to Do Its Job

Fevers are the body's natural defense against viruses and bacteria and help your body fight off an infection. Taking decongestants (afrin, sudafed, neo-synephrine), fever reducers (ibuprofen, acetaminophen), and cough suppressants (dextromethorphan) only suppresses the body's natural defenses. However, high fevers can cause fever-induced seizures in infants and small children. Fever reduction is often needed in fevers 101.5°F or higher in infants over 2 months old to prevent fever induced seizures.

An infant under two months old with a fever over 101°F should go to the emergency room and/or you should call your physician, if available. Call your physician if an infant's fever persists over 24 hours or is higher than 101°F.

Colds and flus are the training ground for the immune system, especially in children. If you don't get sick once in a while, your immune system won't get to make memory immune cells to fight off bugs in the future.

Call Your Physician if:

- Your symptoms get worse
- Your symptoms last a long time (over 10-14 days)
- After feeling a little better, you show signs of a more serious problem: sick-to-your-stomach feeling, vomiting, high fever, shaking, chills, chest pain, or coughing with thick, yellow-green mucus, severe neck or back pain

Call Your Child's Physician if:

- Your child has a persistent (over 3-5 days) cough, sore throat, or ear pain
- Your child's fever lasts longer than 48 hours
- Your infant (less than 1 year) loses his appetite and refuses several feedings
- Your infant doesn't have a wet diaper in more than 8 hours
- Your infant seems overly irritable, or is unusually sleepy, or hard to awaken
- Your infant is less than three months old with a rectal temperature higher than 100.5°F

Post-Infection Immune Support

During the first few days of a cold or flu, people are motivated to stimulate and support their immune system. However, most people stop supporting their immune system way too early because they start to feel better. The risks of not providing immune support (diet, supplements, hydrotherapy, and eliminating immune suppressive activities) during this critical recovery time is an increased susceptibility to catching another virus, contracting a secondary bacterial infection, lingering fatigue, cough, and/or nasal congestion. The recovery stage usually lasts a week after the acute infection is over.

After the acute symptoms of fever, body ache, stomach ache, diarrhea, and lethargy are over, coughs and nasal congestion can linger for weeks if the immune system is not properly supported. Beyond the discomfort of these symptoms, prolonged congestion can increase the risk of contracting a bacterial infection secondary to the earlier viral infection. Secondary bacterial infections are common in individuals who are prone to sinus infections. Increased nasal congestion prevents the sinuses from emptying and provides a prime environment for bacterial growth. A common scenario is increased fatigue, slight facial pain or headache, and slight fever after several days of improvement. At this point ramping up your defenses is crucial to avoid prolonged recovery from a secondary infection.

Change Your Defense Strategy

During the recovery phase of an illness it is important to change your defense strategy. If you suspect a secondary bacterial infection, switch to using anti-bacterial herbs such as goldenseal or usnea (See anti-bacterial herb section in *Chapter 6 Immune Botanicals)* and call your naturopathic physician for proper diagnosis. For lingering cough or fatigue add lomatium or usnea to your defense team. For continued nasal congestion, perform daily *nasal irrigation.* (See Chapter 8 *Hydrotherapy and Topical Treatments)*

In general taking immune supportive herbs (astragalus, ashwagandha, licorice, and american ginseng) for a few weeks after an illness can improve energy, strengthen the immune system, and prevent further complications. *Contrast hydrotherapy* is also an easy immune and circulation boost post infection to add to your daily routine (See Chapter 8 *Hydrotherapy and Topical Treatments).*

Proper Use of Antibiotics

Antibiotics should only be taken for a bacterial infection. They should not be taken for a viral illness, as they are useless in treating viral illnesses and increase antibiotic resistance.

For bacterial infections, it is best to use antibiotics only when all other avenues have been exhausted and in conjunction with good immune support through vitamins, minerals, herbs, and an acidophilus replacement or pro-biotic.

Pro-biotics

Always take an acidophilus supplement when taking antibiotics.

Pro-biotics repopulate the friendly bacteria and can help prevent side effects such as yeast overgrowth and nutrient loss. It is best to take probiotics in between antibiotic doses and for at least a month after finishing the antibiotics. Always buy acidophilus products that are refrigerated to ensure "active" healthy bacteria to restore healthy gut flora.

Pro-biotics have been identified as immune stimulating in the digestive tract. Since 50% of the immune system resides in the digestive tract, probiotics are a great way to support the immune system, especially if there have been frequent antibiotic uses in the past.

Sample Immune Boosting Plans

Common Cold

1000 mg vitamin C every 2 hours (to bowel tolerance)

Avoid all immune suppressing activities

Tea, tincture, or capsules containing: ganoderma, osha, echinacea, thyme, grapefruit seed extract

Eat foods high in vitamins and minerals (*Ginger Soup*)

Ferrum phos 30C homeopathic 3 pellets three times a day

Warming Body or *Warming Sock* Treatment

Nasal Irrigation if nose is congested

Contact with a sick person and under constant stress

Tea, tincture, capsules containing: licorice, ashwagandha, astragalus, asian mushrooms, asian or american ginseng (1-2 doses three times a day)

Vitamin C 1000 mg three times a day

Eat whole foods and avoid sugar

Over 50 years / Get sick often and sickness lingers

Avoid immune suppressive activities

Zinc supplement 30-50 mg a day

Vitamin C 1000 mg three times a day

Tea, tincture, or capsules containing: ganoderma, ashwagandha, holy basil, echinacea, schisandra

Test DHEA levels (blood or saliva)

Warming Sock or *Warming Body* Treatment

Child with a sore throat, mild fever, muscle aches

Decrease sugar and mucous containing foods

Carrot poultice to neck

Glycerite tincture containing: elder flower, chamomile, lemon balm, echinacea, astragalus, goldenseal.

Children's Emergen C 500 mg 2-3 times a day

Warm bath with Epsom salt and 10 drops of lavender essential oil

What About the Flu Vaccine?

Every year, scientists make different flu vaccines because the strains of the influenza virus change yearly. Before the flu season begins, they prepare a new vaccine based on the viruses expected to circulate in the following winter. If they guess right, the vaccine is effective. However, if different strains are circulating, the vaccine provides no benefit and can actually cause harm due to the mercury it contains.

The flu vaccine is one of the only vaccines still containing "thimerosol," a mercury containing product. Mercury may cause neuro-developmental disorders such as autism, attention deficit hyperactivity disorder (ADHD), and speech or language delay in children. Thimerosal is found in multi-use vials. If you want to get the flu vaccine, ask for thimerosal free in single use vials or nasal spray. For more information regarding vaccines, visit the National Vaccine Information Center http://www.nvic.org.

Who Should Get a Flu Shot?

- people 65 or older with a depleted immune system
- nursing home patients
- people with asthma, or long-term diseases (such as HIV or heart disease, chronic lung disease)

- As for children, it is a parent's decision whether to give the vaccine by looking at the risk/benefit ratio for their children. The death rate in children from flu is virtually zero, while mercury can have severe effects on a developing brain.

Who Might Not Be Able to Get a Flu Shot?

- people with certain allergies, especially to eggs
- people who have an illness, such as pneumonia
- people with a high fever
- pregnant women

Side Effects

- soreness at the site of the vaccination.
- fever, tiredness, and sore muscles.
- serious allergic reaction if you have an egg allergy (the vaccine is grown in chicken eggs)
- Guillain-Barre syndrome: debilitating neurological disorder

---

[1] Predy, GN. (2005). Efficacy of an extract of North American ginseng containing poly-furanosyl-pyranosyl-saccharides for preventing upper respiratory tract infections: a randomized controlled trial. *CMAJ*. Oct 25; 173(9):1043-8.

[2]Tierra, L. (2000). *A kid's herb book*. San Francisco, CA: Robert. R. Reed Publishing.

[3] Tierra, L. (2000). *A kid's herb book*. San Francisco, CA: Robert. R. Reed Publishing.

[4] Tierra, L. (2000). *A kid's herb book*. San Francisco, CA: Robert. R. Reed Publishing.

8 | Hydrotherapy and Topical Treatments

Hydrotherapy for Immune Stimulation

The use of water in healing dates back to the first medical records of Hippocrates. Hydrotherapy, which means "water therapy," involves the use of hot and cold applications of water to the body. Hydrotherapy is beneficial:

- to stimulate removal of toxins and waste
- to strengthen the digestive system
- to stimulate the immune and metabolic systems
- to improve circulation
- to increase overall tonification of the body

Hydrotherapy stimulates the immune system and fights infections in two ways. It increases the amount of blood flow to specific areas of the body and it stimulates immune cells in the digestive tract and thymus gland.

In particular, the *Warming Sock* treatment acts to reflexively increase circulation and decrease congestion in the upper respiratory passages, the head, and throat. The *Warming Body* treatment stimulates the thymus gland and supports healthy digestive function. This treatment is also effective for pain relief and increases the healing response during acute infections. Both treatments have a sedating action and many people report they sleep much better during or after the treatment.

Warming Sock Treatment

This treatment is best if repeated for three nights in a row, or as instructed by your physician. It is indicated for sore throat or any inflammation or infection of the throat, neck pain, ear infections, headaches, migraines, nasal congestion, upper respiratory infections, coughs, bronchitis, and sinus infections.

Contraindications for Warming Sock Treatment

Use this treatment with caution if you have diabetes, Raynaud's phenomenon or syndrome, arterial insufficiency or advanced intermittent claudication. The warming phase is especially important for these patients. Please consult your physician.

Supplies

1 pair white cotton socks (colored socks can bleed onto the skin)
1 pair thick wool socks
Towel
Warm bath or warm foot bath

Directions

1. Soak the cotton socks completely in cold water. Wring
    them out thoroughly so they do not drip.

2. Thoroughly warm your feet by soaking in warm water
    for at least 5-10 minutes or by taking a warm bath for 5-
    10 minutes. This is very important! The treatment will
    not be as effective and could be harmful if your feet are
    not warmed first.

3. Dry off your feet and body with a dry towel.

4. Place the cold, wet cotton socks on your feet.
    Immediately pull the thick wool socks over the wet
    socks.

5. Go directly to bed. Avoid getting chilled.

6. Keep the socks on overnight. You will find the wet
    cotton socks will be dry in the morning.

Warming Body Treatment

The goal of this treatment is to artificially induce a fever
by increasing the body core temperature. This stimulates
the immune system and assists in destroying heat sensitive
viruses/bacteria, as well as promoting detoxification and
elimination through the skin (via sweating).

Contraindications for Warming Body Treatment

Do not use this treatment if you have any of the
following conditions: serious illness or decreased vitality
(elderly or very young children), pre-existing high fever,
tachycardia, arrhythmia, other cardiac deficiency
conditions, open wounds or active bleeding, pulmonary

deficiency, respiratory insufficiency, lupus, acute high
blood pressure, diabetes, pregnancy, breast feeding, or
multiple sclerosis.

Supplies

> Bathtub or tub full of hot water (hot but not burning)
> Towels or a flannel sheet
> Two wool blankets
> Hot water bottle or heating pad
> Drinking water

Directions

1. Make sure someone else is at home with you for the treatment duration.
2. Immerse as much of your body as possible in the tub for five minutes.
3. Immediately dry off, dress warmly and get into a bed or couch lined with towels or a flannel sheet, with at least two wool blankets on top.
4. Place a hot water bottle or heating pad over the upper abdomen (over the liver, stomach, and spleen).
5. Sweat for at least twenty minutes. Drink plenty of water during your sweat so you'll remain hydrated.
6. After the sweat, have some broth, soup, or vegetable juice to help replenish electrolyte minerals lost during the sweating process.
7. Make sure to dry off completely and dress in warm dry clothes to prevent getting chilled after the sweat.

Contrast Hydrotherapy

Contrast hydrotherapy is the application of hot and cold water to the body to boost the immune system by increasing circulation throughout the body and to stimulate the thymus gland. Contrast hydrotherapy can also keep you warmer during cold winter days by stimulating circulation throughout the entire body. It is recommended to use during the recovery period after an infection and daily during the cold winter months as a preventative measure.

Contrast hydrotherapy has been traditionally used in Sweden and Finland as part of the sauna tradition. Participants will sit in a hot sauna and then jump in a cold river. This process is repeated several times to obtain the desired results. A milder version is to end a shower with a cycle of hot and cold water.

Directions

1. Check water heater is set to 120^0F or less.
2. Take a hot shower for at least 5 minutes.
3. Once the body is heated, switch to the coldest water tolerable and rinse the whole body including the torso for at least 15-30 seconds.
4. Switch the water to the hottest temperature for 2-3 minutes and then repeat step 2.
5. If desired repeat the cycle again ending with cold and then dry off. Gradually increase the length of time exposed to cold and gradually decrease temperature of cold water used.

Nasal Irrigation[1]

Nasal irrigation is an internal cleansing of the nasal passages useful in decreasing nasal congestion, allergies, sinus infections, colds, and many other ailments. The dust, dirt, pollen, bacteria, viruses, and smoke that gets trapped by the nasal mucosa can easily be washed away by this simple procedure. In addition, the salt water will kill bacteria in the nasal passage and decrease congestion to effectively treat sinus infections and to prevent colds and flus from developing into sinus infections.

Supplies

Porcelain neti pots made specifically for the nasal wash are available. Alternatively, a small regular tea pot may be used.

16 ounces of warm, clean, filtered water free of contaminants or distilled water

Non –iodized salt

Direction:

1. Pour 8 ounces of clean, filtered warm water into the pot. Water that is too cool may increase congestion, while water that is too warm may cause irritation of the delicate lining of the nose.

2. Stir pure, non-iodized salt into the water until it is completely dissolved. The amount depends on how finely ground the salt is. Use ¼ teaspoon with finely ground salt such as table salt, or ½ teaspoon with coarse varieties like kosher salt or sea salt. The resulting saline solution should not burn.

3. Lean over the sink so that you are looking directly into the basin, then rotate your head to the side so that one nostril is directly above the other. The forehead should remain level with the chin or slightly higher. Insert the spout into the upper nostril until it makes a comfortable seal. Keeping your mouth open, pour the solution into the upper nostril and let it drain out through the lower. You should be able to breathe comfortably through your mouth. If the solution drains into your mouth, lower your forehead in relation to your chin. Continue pouring until the pot is empty.

4. Exhale vigorously through your nose to clear excess mucus and water. Quickly draw the abdomen toward the spine during each exhalation. If using a tissue, be sure not to pinch the nostrils closed. Continue until they are both clear.

5. Mix another batch of saline in the pot and repeat the procedure on the other side, again exhaling vigorously to clear the nasal passages.

6. After irrigating both nostrils, both nasal passages should feel soothed with increased air-flow through both nostrils.

Mustard Pack

A mustard pack can be applied externally to the chest for colds or coughs. Mustard and mustard oils are absorbed into the skin and act deep in the lung to encourage expectoration, or the loosening of mucus. It is especially helpful in conditions with a tight chest and a dry cough. Mustard is also anti-bacterial and can help eliminate lung infection in addition to its clearing effects. In addition to skin absorption, this mustard application will also give off a mild aroma, which has therapeutic effects as you breathe in.

CAUTION should be used when applying mustard. It can be irritating to the skin and the pack should be removed if you experience pain or notice a glowing redness on the skin. Avoid contact with this preparation on sensitive tissues including the nipples, genitals, face, and especially eyes. For children, do not leave application on for longer than 10 minutes and for adults no longer than 15-20 minutes. For sensitive individuals, patch test the mixture before applying to a larger part of the skin for at least 10-15 minutes. Remove immediately if noticing irritation and wash with soap and water.

Supplies

7. 1-2 Tb dry mustard
8. 1 cup white flour
9. Cotton cloth (12" x 12") - old T-shirt, cheesecloth, etc.
10. Plastic wrap
11. Hot water bottle or hot gel pack

Directions

1. Have the patient wear a robe and lie down comfortably.
2. Combine 1-2 Tb of dry mustard (depending on its freshness or potency) and 1 cup of flour in a small mixing bowl.
3. Add enough hot water to make a paste, pouring water a little at a time.
4. Spread mustard/flour paste about 1/2 in thick over a cotton cloth or piece of cheesecloth. Cover the paste with another piece of cloth to make a "mustard sandwich".
5. Place the pack on the bare chest area and cover it with a sheet of plastic wrap. Place either a hot water bottle or hot gel pack on top of the plastic wrap.
6. Leave on no longer than 10 minutes for children or 15-20 minutes for adults.
7. Remove the pack and discard it.
8. The patient should wipe off the chest with a warm wash cloth. If needed, repeat the pack twice a day to encourage clearing of congestion from the chest.

Homemade Vapor Rub

Vapor rub is most effective at opening congested nasal and sinus passages, thus clearing congestion in the upper airways.

1. Combine 20 drops essential oils (any combination of eucalyptus, hyssop, thyme, peppermint, or basil) with 2 oz. almond or olive oil.

2. Rub the oil mixture on the chest area to relieve chest congestion or apply to a cotton ball you can sniff to open the nasal and sinus passages.

Carrot Poultice

Carrot poultice is very helpful in decreasing painful sore throats. It has especially good results in children under six years old, but also works for older children and adults. A carrot poultice can be made either hot or cold, depending on which feels best.

Contraindications

Carrot allergy or sensitivity, open wounds

Supplies

One large carrot
Cotton cloth (12" x 12") handkerchief, cheesecloth, etc.
Wool scarf
Plastic wrap
Crushed ice (if cold poultice)
Hot water bottle (if hot poultice)
For a cold poultice, combine ice with the carrot.
For a hot poultice, place cloth and carrot packet in hot water and squeeze out excess water before applying to neck, or alternatively, apply a hot water bottle over the poultice.

Directions

1. Grate a large carrot into the center one-third of the cotton cloth. For a cold poultice, combine about 1 cup crushed ice with the carrot.

2. Fold the other two-thirds of the cotton cloth over the carrot, creating a packet (with one thickness of cloth under the carrot). For a hot poultice, place packet in hot water and then gently squeeze out excess water (or you can just use hot water bottle).

3. Apply the single thickness side of the carrot packet to the front of the neck and cover with plastic wrap (just over the packet).

4. Wrap the wool scarf gently around the neck and fasten in place. For a hot poultice, apply a hot water bottle or gel pack over the scarf.

5. Leave poultice in place for a minimum of 30 minutes.

Note: Do not wrap the cloth or scarf around the neck too tightly. It should be firmly against the skin but loose enough to insert a finger between the cloth and neck.

Garlic Feet

This is a classic treatment for stubborn coughs and infections in the lungs or upper airways. Garlic is a strong anti-bacterial and anti-viral with potent aromatic compounds easily absorbed through the skin, into the blood and then into the lungs.[2] A garlic treatment is specifically indicated for symptoms of clear to white mucus with a cold body reaction. Garlic applied to the skin will quickly show up in the breath.

This treatment should not be used on someone with a garlic allergy or impaired sensation in the feet (like peripheral neuropathy). You should also prepare yourself and your family for the whole house (and the patient) smelling like garlic. Chewing on a few sprigs of parsley or taking chlorophyll capsules can decrease the smell of garlic on your breath.

Directions

1. Mince 2-3 garlic cloves and mix with 1-2 Tb olive oil.

2. Split the mixture in half and wrap each half in a small cotton cloth or cheesecloth with two or three layers of folded cloth between the mixture and the sole of the foot.

3. Tape one garlic pack to the sole of each foot with athletic tape or bandage tape. *If you have significant congestion in the lungs, apply the wrapped mixture to your chest. This is also very effective and a more direct treatment.*

4. Leave on the feet for 1 hour or overnight (Must be lying down).

5. Repeat nightly as needed to clear the lungs and upper airways of congestion.

Note: People with sensitive skin may notice irritation and should place a layer of olive oil on the soles of the feet before taping the cloth to the feet and only use for one hour. If too much irritation develops, rinse off immediately with soap and water.

[1] Himalayan International Institute of Yoga Science and Philosophy. (1994). *Neti Pot*. Honesdale, PA.

[2] Tierra, L. (2000). *A kid's herb book*. San Francisco, CA: Robert. R. Reed Publishing.

9 | Recipes for Immune Health

Hot Foods for Colds

If you have cold reactions such as slight fever with many chills, cold skin and feet, and diarrhea, try using "hot" foods. These foods contain substances called "mucolytics" (similar to over-the-counter expectorant cough syrups) which can liquefy thick mucus accumulated in the sinuses and breathing passages. Enjoy these hot foods freely:

- chili peppers
- hot mustard
- radishes
- black pepper
- onions
- garlic
- horseradish (wasabi)

Teas

Dr. Christensen's Spicy Immune Tea

Mix together:

¼ cup of the following herbs: astragalus root, echinacea root, licorice root, ashwagandha root, schisandra berries

1/8 cup fresh chopped ginger root.

2 organic cinnamon sticks (broken into small pieces) and/or
    1/8 cup dried orange peel and/or 1 tsp cloves

Place 1-2 Tb of the mixture in a small sauce pan and add 1-2
cups water. Bring to a boil, reduce heat and simmer, covered, for
15 minutes. Cool slightly and strain. Sweeten with stevia or
honey if desired. Drink straight or with a bit of milk or cream. 1-
2 cups per day

Clear Your Throat[1]

    1 lemon
    2 cups water
    1/16-1/8 tsp cayenne powder

Squeeze lemon into water. Add cayenne powder and sweeten
with honey to taste. Drink throughout the day.

Dr. Mary Bove's Immune Herbal Punch[2]

    Mix ½ cup of the following herbs: chamomile, elder flowers,
    lemon balm, nettles, red clover and spearmint.

Use 1Tb per cup of boiling water for adults and 1 Tb per 2 cups
of boiling water for children. Steep, covered, for 15 minutes and
then strain. Mix with 2 cups of juice. Kids can drink 1 8oz cup a
day and adults 2-3 8 oz. cups a day.

Sneeze Tea[3]

Sneeze tea is great for sneezing caused by allergies or illness.

    Mix ½ cup of the following herbs: elder flowers, yarrow, and
    echinacea.

Steep one tablespoon per cup of boiling water, covered, for 20
minutes. Drink ¼ to ½ cup every two hours.

Ginger-ale Fizz

Ginger-ale Fizz is a great way to stay hydrated and to treat
nausea. This recipe is adapted from Lesley Tierra's recipe[4].

   1 tsp fresh ginger or ½ tsp of ginger powder
   1 tsp lemon balm and/or chamomile (optional)
   1 cup water
   ½ cup carbonated water
   1 tsp honey or a pinch of stevia

Add the ginger to 1 cup water in saucepan and simmer for 5
minutes. Remove from heat and add lemon balm and chamomile
to steep for 10 minutes covered. Add the carbonated water and
sweetener to taste. Sip 1 to 2 Tb every few minutes to relieve
nausea.

Syrups

   Syrups are a great way for kids to take herbs and to
soothe sore throats and coughs. Licorice, ginger, garlic,
elder flower or berry, lemon balm, cinnamon, fennel, and
cayenne work well in syrups.

Onion Syrup[5]

Onion syrup is a natural antibiotic and can treat mucus
congestion, coughs, bronchitis, colds, and flu.

   1 medium minced onion
   lemon juice
   3 Tb honey
   1/8 tsp cayenne

Put the onion in a saucepan with enough lemon juice to cover.
Add 2 cups water and simmer for 20 minutes. Blend in a food

processor or blender. Stir in honey and cayenne. Take 1 tsp several times a day or as needed. Store in the refrigerator.

Throat Coat

Throat coat is best used for sore throats which feel better with warm drinks.

¼ cup licorice root
1/8 cup fresh ginger root
1/8 cup slippery elm root
pinch of cayenne
½ cup honey or glycerin

Boil the 3 roots in 2 cups of water for 15 to 20 minutes. Strain while warm and add a cayenne and honey or glycerin. Stir well until dissolved. Cool and place in a jar to refrigerate. The syrup keeps for one month if refrigerated. Take 1 tsp every hour to soothe the throat and stimulate the immune system.

Blasted Cough Syrup

This is a modified version of Lesley Tierra's Garlic Syrup[6]. It is specific for stubborn coughs, bronchitis, pneumonia, and clear to white mucus with cold reaction symptoms.

½ cup lemon juice
½ cup water
5 large cloves of garlic minced or pressed
1 tsp grated ginger or ¼ tsp ginger powder
dash of cayenne
2 Tb thyme
½ cup honey

Boil the water and steep the thyme for 20 minutes covered. Add the rest of the ingredients and blend in a food processor or blender. Take 1 tsp every 2 hours as needed to address the cough.

Vinegars

Winter Tonic Cider

This is a modified version of Snappy Winter Cider.[7]

¼ cup onions
¼ cup garlic
¼ cup ginger
3 Tb horseradish
3 Tb mustard seed
3 Tb black pepper
1-2 cayenne pods
apple cider vinegar
honey or glycerine

Mix vegetables and herbs with the cayenne pods in a glass container with a lid. Pour apple cider vinegar over the herbs and cover them by one inch. Cover the container and shake daily for two weeks. Strain and add one part honey or glycerine to three parts vinegar. Take ½ tsp to 1 tsp every hour when feeling a sore throat or the beginning of a cold.

Breakfast

Immune Boosting Smoothie

2 cups milk or soy or rice beverage
1 cup plain nonfat yogurt
1 serving of a multivitamin supplement (capsules or liquid
    preferred)

one frozen banana, cut up
1/2 cup frozen blueberries
1/2 cup each of your favorite fruit, frozen (e.g., organic
  strawberries, papaya, mango)
1 Tb flax oil or 2 Tb flaxseed meal
3 oz. tofu
1 serving whey, or vegan protein powder (optional)
2 Tb peanut butter (optional)

Combine all ingredients and blend until smooth. Serve immediately after blending while the mixture still has a bubbly, milkshake-like consistency. Serves 2.

Hearty Breakfast Bread

The recipe is modified from Mountain Bread recipe from A Taste of History[8]. It is full of B vitamins, essential fatty acids, and healthy protein to keep you going all morning.

4 cups whole wheat flour
1 cup water
1 cup honey
1/3 cup wheat germ
1/3 cup olive oil or canola oil
¼ cup sesame seeds
¼ cup chopped walnuts or pecans
¼ cup molasses
2 Tb dry milk
1 ½ tsp baking powder
1 ½ tsp salt

Mix all ingredients together until smooth. Pour into a 8 x 8x2 inch lightly greased pan. Bake at 300^0F for 1 hour or until bread pulls away from the sides. Let stand overnight to dry and store in a plastic bag. Bread will be firm.

Dr. Milliman's Immune Support Breakfast

The immune support breakfast was designed by Dr. Milliman, a naturopathic doctor, to support the immune system and overall health. The immune support breakfast is also a great way to lower cholesterol, increase fiber, and have an adequate amount of non-animal protein for breakfast. The pumpkin seeds and other nuts are high in zinc, calcium, magnesium, copper, and iron. Sunflower seeds are particularly high in selenium.

Milk thistle is a seed that protects the liver against damage by toxins, infection, or other stressors. Milk thistle also aids in decreasing inflammation and high cholesterol through its action on the liver.

Flax seeds provide fiber and omega-3 fatty acids to decrease constipation and decrease inflammation in the body. The omega-3 oil found in flax seeds is protective against cardiovascular disease, cancer, autoimmune conditions, and skin disorders.

If you have food allergies or sensitivities, please substitute appropriate food groups to modify the recipe. For example, if you have allergies to almonds, use cashews. If you are allergic to gluten, substitute rice bran for the oat bran and use a nutty puffed rice cereal instead of grains.

When purchasing ingredients, in all cases, fresh is preferred to frozen and frozen is preferred to canned. When purchasing seeds, buying organic is especially important. Many non-organic seeds are coated with an anti-fungal

agent called captan. It's especially toxic and usually
appears as a pink-colored residue on seeds.

>4 cups Rolled Grains: 2 cups rolled oats (flakes) plus 2 cups
>of some other available grain (rye, barley, rolled rice
>flakes, etc.). Use 4 cups rolled oats if other grains are
>unavailable. *Choose only grains edible after soaking—
>no cooking of the foods in this recipe is done, on purpose.*
>2 cups Oat Bran (use rice bran if gluten-sensitive)
>1 cups Organic Fruits (fresh, dried, frozen) preservative free
>raisins, dates, blueberries, strawberries, etc.
>1 cup Sunflower and/or Pumpkin Seeds (ground)
>1 cup Nuts (raw, chopped, unsalted) Begin with walnuts and
>almonds
>1 cup Lecithin Granules
>1 cup Ground Flax Seed *
>1 cup Milk Thistle Seeds * (Silybum marianum), optional
>
>3 tsp spice blend or other spices to taste: try coriander, fennel,
>turmeric, ginger, cinnamon, cardamom, nutmeg, "apple
>pie" or "pumpkin pie" blends
>*Flax and milk thistle seeds are available at most health
>food stores. Grind them in a coffee grinder/blender/food
>processor.

Combine all ingredients and keep in refrigerator. Soak ½ cup of
the mixture for 30 minutes or longer before eating (i.e.
overnight) or mix with plain yogurt. For soaking, use water, soy
milk, rice milk, nut milk, apple juice, etc.

Egg-Free French Toast

This modern twist on an old favorite is great for people with egg allergies or who are trying to lower cholesterol. It is modified from Chris Cavanaugh's recipe[9].

1 cup silken tofu
1 cup almond milk, nonfat milk, soy milk, or rice milk
1/2 tsp ground cinnamon
1/2 tsp ground ginger
4 slices whole grain bread or sprouted grain bread

In a blender, puree tofu and milk. Add cinnamon and ginger. Heat skillet coated with oil over medium-high heat. Dip bread in mixture, soaking both sides. Cook in skillet until browned on both sides, about 5 minutes. Drizzle with honey.

Soups

Hearty Vegetable Soup

This tasty vegetable soup is wonderful for relieving sinus congestion, supporting the immune system, and relieving diarrhea.[10] Serves 8-10.

8-10 cups vegetable broth or water
8 cloves garlic, peeled and chopped
8 carrots, chopped
2 potatoes, chopped
2 onions, chopped
¼ cup fresh lovage root, chopped
2 fresh burdock roots, chopped
1/8 cup dried astragalus root, chopped
½ cup barley
¼ cup quinoa
10-12 calendula flowers

Combine water, vegetable broth, vegetables, and roots. Bring to a boil over medium heat. Gently boil for 2-3 hours, adding more water if necessary. Reduce heat to simmer and add barley, quinoa and calendula, cooking for 45-60 minutes more. Enjoy with whole grain bread or crackers.

Coconut Chicken Soup

Coconut chicken soup is a great twist on chicken noodle soup. The wonderful flavors of ginger, garlic, astragalus, and shitake mushrooms provide powerful support for the immune system. Serves 4.

2 Tb finely chopped ginger

1/8 cup astragalus root (optional)
¼ cup chopped cilantro
½ tsp pepper
3 Tb chopped garlic
½ cup chopped red onion
5 fresh or dried shitake mushrooms thinly sliced (if dried,
       soak in hot water for 10-15 minutes to soften)
2 cans (14 oz) unsweetened coconut milk
2 cups chicken stock
8 oz chicken breasts cut into strips
5 Tb fresh lime juice
3 Tb Asian fish sauce
½ tsp of cayenne
Salt to taste

Combine ginger, astragalus, cilantro, pepper, garlic, onion, coconut milk, and chicken stock. Simmer for 10 minutes. Add chicken and simmer for 10-15 more minutes. Take the soup off the heat and let cool for a minute or two before adding the lime juice, fish sauce, cayenne, and salt to taste. Eat alone or with brown rice.

Cream of Pumpkin Soup[11]

This delicious squash soup is high in beta carotene and full of garlic, ginger, and cayenne to boost the immune system and blast any cold or flu away.

2 ½ lbs. fresh pumpkin (or butternut squash) peeled and cut
       into 2 inch cubes
4 ½ cups chicken broth
3 Tb unsweetened butter
1 cup finely chopped leeks, white part only
3 large cloves garlic, crushed

1 tsp curry powder
2 tsp ground ginger
1 ½ tsp ground coriander
2 tsp paprika
2 cans (14 oz) unsweetened coconut milk
2 Tb soy sauce
½ cup fresh cilantro, chopped
Salt to taste

Combine the pumpkin and chicken broth in a large heavy pot and bring to a boil over medium heat. Cook covered until the pumpkin is tender. Puree the pumpkin and liquid in a blender until smooth. Sauté the leeks in butter until soft. Add garlic, curry power, ginger, coriander, and paprika to the leeks. Cook stirring over low heat, for two minutes. Add the coconut milk, bring to a boil and simmer for five minutes. Stir in the pureed pumpkin and cook for five more minutes. Remove from heat and stir in the soy sauce, cilantro, and salt to taste.

Thai Carrot Bisque

The recipe is also called Tom Yum Carrot Soup in Thailand. The recipe is adapted from Rebecca Christensen's Thai Carrot Bisque. It is an extremely flavorful way to eat lots of carrots full of beta-carotene. Serves 6-8.

2 Tb vegetable oil
2 Tb honey or stevia equivalent
4 cups vegetable stock
2 Tb minced fresh ginger
2 cups yellow onion, coarsely chopped
4 cups carrots, coarsely chopped
1 can (14oz) coconut milk
2 tsp salt

3-4 cloves garlic
¼ cup fresh lime juice
cayenne pepper to taste
Garnish: cilantro, 1 tablespoon cream or flax oil per cup,
    croutons.

In a large pot, sauté the onions, salt, honey or substitute for 5 minutes until the onions are soft and fragrant. Add the carrots, ginger, lime juice, vegetable stock and coconut milk and simmer for 20-30 minutes. Puree the soup in a blender or food processor until smooth. Garnish with cilantro, cream or flax oil and croutons. Serve immediately.

Sweet Potato Soup

The recipe is modified from Cooking Live.[12] The spices can be adjusted to vary the taste of the soup. Serves 2-3.

1 Tb flour or corn starch
1 Tb unsalted butter
1 1/2 cups chicken broth (or vegetable broth, if desired)
1 Tb honey
1 1/2 cups cooked sweet potatoes
1/2 tsp ground ginger
½ tsp cayenne powder
1/8 tsp ground cinnamon
1/8 tsp ground nutmeg
1 cup milk (cow, almond, rice, soy)
Salt

In a heavy saucepot, over medium-low heat, cook the flour and butter, stirring constantly until roux achieves a light caramel color. Add the broth and honey, bring to a boil, then lower to a simmer. Stir in the sweet potatoes and spices, bring to a simmer again, and cook for 5 minutes more. In a blender, puree the soup in batches and return to saucepot. Add the milk and reheat soup. Season with salt and pepper, ladle into warm soup bowls and serve.

Gazpacho

Gazpacho is a cold soup chock full of immune boosting herbs and spices. Gazpacho is best enjoyed during the summer, but can be a great warming soup with the addition of ginger in the winter. Serves 2-3.

> 4-5 roma tomatoes or 2-3 medium tomatoes, cubed
> 1 cucumber, peeled and cubed
> 1 small sweet onion, chopped
> 1 cup fresh basil, chopped
> 1-2 cloves garlic, minced
> 2 Tb organic extra-virgin olive oil
> ¼ cup parsley, chopped
> ¼ cup pine nuts
> ¼ cup walnuts
> 1-2 tsp sea salt to taste
> Black pepper and cayenne pepper to taste
> 1-2 Tb ginger, minced (during the winter)

In a food processor or blender, blend all ingredients except salt, pepper, and cayenne. Add spices to taste and enjoy with sprouted bread, whole grain crackers, or top with toasted pumpkin seeds for added zinc.

Salads

Quinoa Salad with Rice and Black Beans

Quinoa salad is high in B vitamins, vegetable protein, and vitamin C. I was introduced to this tasty recipe from my friend Sally Horrobin.

½ cup quinoa
1 14 oz can of vegetable broth
1 ½ tsp ground cumin
½ cup water
½ cup short grain brown rice
1 can (14 oz) black beans, rinsed and drained
2 green onions, sliced thinly
1 red pepper, diced
2 plum tomatoes, diced
½ cup corn
¼ cup cilantro, minced
4 Tb lime juice
2 Tb olive oil
¼ tsp salt, ground black pepper to taste
1/8 tsp cayenne

Put quinoa in a fine sieve and rinse well. Combine quinoa, 1 cup vegetable broth, and ½ tsp of cumin in a sauce pan. Bring to a boil and then reduce heat to cook for 15 to 20 minutes, until the broth has been absorbed. Combine the remaining broth with enough water to make one cup in a second pan and add the rice and ½ tsp cumin. Bring to a boil until the water just covers the rice. Cook covered another 15 minutes. Combine quinoa and rice in a large bowl. Add black beans, green onions, bell pepper, tomatoes, corn, and cilantro. Put lime juice, olive oil, and remaining 1/2 tsp cumin, salt, black pepper and cayenne in a jar. Shake and pour it over the salad. Serve immediately. Serves 6.

Crunchy Salad[13]

    2 cups cauliflower florets
    1/2 cup grape tomatoes
    4 Tb red bell pepper, diced
    2 Tb finely chopped cilantro
    2 Tb chopped scallion
    2 Tb lemon juice
    4 tsp olive oil
    4 Tb feta or goat cheese, crumbled
    Salt to taste

In a medium bowl, combine all the vegetables. Mix the lemon juice and olive oil and pour over the vegetable mixture. Salt to taste and sprinkle cheese on top before serving. Serves 2.

Mexican Bean Salsa

This is a family favorite my mother would always make. It is easy to prepare and tastes even better as leftovers. It's a perfect way to get kids to eat vegetables and you can serve it with chips like a salsa or as a salad.

    2 cans black beans
    1 can pinto beans
    1 can kidney or white beans
    1 green pepper, diced
    1 onion, diced
    1 can (14 oz) olives
    2 cups corn
    ¾ cup balsamic vinegar
    3-4 cans diced tomatoes

2-3 cloves garlic, minced
Mexican seasoning to taste
¼ tsp cayenne (optional)

Mix all ingredients together in a large bowl. Season to taste with Mexican seasonings and add cayenne, if desired. Serves 6-10.

Beets and Goat Cheese Salad

The recipe is adapted from Cynthia Lair's Luscious Beet Salad and is a favorite at most gatherings.

4 large beets
1 bunch beet greens (optional)
¼ cup toasted pumpkin seeds
2 scallions, finely chopped
¼ lb. goat or feta cheese
3 Tb extra-virgin olive oil
2 Tb balsamic vinegar
¼ tsp Dijon mustard
¼ tsp ground pepper
1 Tb basil, finely chopped
1 tsp fresh thyme, finely chopped
1 tsp fresh peppermint leaves, finely chopped

Wash beets and remove tops. Place beets in a large pot with water and simmer until beets are tender (about an hour). Drain the water and cool.

Toast pumpkin seeds by placing in a skillet over medium heat. Gently move the skillet back and forth while stirring the pumpkin seeds to toast evenly. Remove the seeds from the heat once they begin to pop and give off a nutty aroma. Wash beet greens and chop into bite sized pieces. Drop into boiling water for 30 seconds and then remove. Mix the oil, vinegar, mustard, pepper, basil, thyme and peppermint leaves in a jar and shake well.

Peel the beets and cut into cubes. Place beets, beet greens, scallions, cheese, and pumpkin seeds in a salad bowl. Pour dressing over the salad and toss gently. Serves 6.

Wild Rice with Toasted Pecans

The recipe is adapted from "Wild Seasons Wild Rice Medley with Toasted Pecans. [14]"

> 1 cup short grain brown rice
> 2 ¼ cups cold water
> ½ cup wild rice
> 1 ½ cups cold water
> ¾ cup broken pecans
> 3/4 cup carrots, chopped
> ¾ cup celery, chopped
> 1 lemon
> 1 Tb lemon zest
> Salt and freshly ground pepper to taste
> 1-2 Tb olive oil

Wash each kind of rice separately and put each into a medium sized pot that has a tight fitting lid, but do not cover. Add the first amount of water to the brown rice and second amount to the wild rice. Place the pots over high heat and after the water reaches a boil, reduce heat to very low. Cover the pots with lids and allow the rice to cook for 35 minutes. Take off the heat and keep covered for another five minutes.

Spoon both kinds of rice into a large bowl and add pecans, carrots, celery, salt, and pepper. Squeeze lemon juice over the mixture. Grate 1 Tb of lemon peel and add to the mixture. Stir well. Serves 4-5.

Main Meals

Vegetarian Lasagna

The recipe is adapted from Food For All Seasons and is a pot-luck favorite.

2 Tb olive or canola oil
1 cup green onions, minced
1 bunch spinach, chopped
10-12 lasagna noodle strips, slightly undercooked
6 cups tomato sauce
1 can black olives
1 cup Portobello or other mushrooms
2 cups refried beans
1 cup tofu mashed with 1 Tb light miso
Salt and finely ground black pepper to taste

Preheat oven to 350^{0}F. Sauté green onions and mushrooms in a skillet with oil. Cook until onions are transparent. Add spinach and cook 2 minutes.

In a large baking dish, layer lasagna strips, tomato sauce, beans, spinach mixture, and tofu mixture until lasagna noodles are used up. Top with tomato sauce. Cover and bake for 20 minutes. Serves 6.

Shitake Chicken

The recipe is adapted from Chis Cavenaugh's recipe[15]

4 oz boneless, skinless, chicken breast, cut into 1-inch strips, seasoned with salt and pepper

1 cup fresh shiitake mushrooms, sliced
¼ tsp dried thyme
¼ tsp dried or fresh rosemary, finely chopped
2 tsp olive oil
2 Tb red wine
Pinch of salt

In a medium nonstick skillet, brown chicken in olive oil. Add remaining ingredients except the red wine. Stir, while browning the shitake mushrooms, for 5 minutes. Add red wine to the skillet and simmer for 2-3 more minutes.

Chicken Pesto Pasta

1/8 cup pine nuts
1/8 tsp salt
1 cup packed basil leaves
¼ cup parsley (optional)
2 cloves garlic peeled
1 Tb olive oil
1 Tb flax oil
1 Tb parmesan, grated (optional)
2 4-oz chicken breasts, grilled and cut into 1 oz strips
3 cups cooked whole grain pasta (wheat, rice or spelt) or high
      protein pasta (lentil)

In a blender or food processor, finely grind pine nuts and salt. Add basil leaves, parsley leaves, and garlic. Blend well. Add oil and process until smooth. Add grated parmesan. Blend well. Toss with cooked pasta and top with chicken. Serves 2-3.

Shrimp Salad Pita

The recipe is adapted from Cavanaugh's[16] recipe. It is high in zinc, protein, vitamin C, and garlic.

5 ounces cooked shrimp, chopped
1 Tb *Healthier Mayonnaise* or mayonnaise
2 Tb celery, diced
2 Tb yellow bell pepper, diced
½ tsp dill, chopped
¼ tsp lemon zest, grated
1/8 tsp garlic, chopped
1 whole-wheat pita
1 cup watercress

Combine shrimp, mayonnaise, celery, dill, lemon zest, and garlic. Stuff into the pita and top with watercress. Serves 1.

Ham Fried Rice

The recipe is a favorite dish given a healthy spin. It is full of beta carotene, vitamin C, protein, garlic, and fiber.

¼ cup olive or canola oil
4 cups cooked brown or white rice
1 cup ham, diced
¾ cup carrots, grated
1 red or yellow bell pepper, diced
1 medium onion, diced
3 cloves garlic, minced
¼ cup Bragg's liquid amino acids or reduced salt soy sauce
1/8 tsp cayenne (optional)
Salt and pepper to taste

Sauté the garlic and onion in the oil using a large skillet on medium heat. Add the ham, carrots, and bell pepper cooking for another 2-3 minutes, stirring often. Add the rice and mix well for 1-2 minutes. Pour the Bragg's amino acid or soy sauce over the mixture, mix well and cook for an additional 3-4 minutes. Add cayenne, salt and pepper to taste. Serves 4.

Lemon-Garlic Grilled Salmon[17]

 5 oz salmon fillet
 1 Tb soy sauce
 1 Tb olive oil
 2 teaspoons fresh ginger, minced
 1 teaspoon garlic, chopped
 ½ teaspoon lemon zest, grated

Combine all ingredients and marinate the salmon fillet in this mixture for 30 minutes (or overnight in the refrigerator for a more distinct taste). Grill until fish flakes easily. Serves 1.

Desserts and Snacks

Cherries Jubilee

 1 cup frozen cherries
 ½ cup frozen cranberries (optional)
 1 cup calcium-enriched vanilla soy milk, rice milk, or almond
  milk
 1 Tb honey
 1/8 teaspoon cinnamon

Combine all ingredients in a blender. Blend on puree setting until smooth. Serves 1.

Mayan Chocolate Shake

This recipe works great as dessert or breakfast. It is high in calcium and protein.

1 medium ripe banana
3/4 cup plain yogurt
2 Tb organic peanut, almond, or cashew butter
1 Tb unsweetened cocoa powder
¾ cup soy, rice, or almond milk (can use chocolate milk if
    you don't have cocoa powder)
1/8 teaspoon cinnamon
1 Tb honey or a pinch of stevia

Combine all ingredients in a blender. Puree for 1 minute until smooth. Serves 2.

Baked Apple Delight[18]

1 Granny Smith apple
2 Tb raisins
1 Tb walnuts, chopped
1/8 teaspoon cinnamon
1 Tb orange juice or apple juice
1-2 Tb vanilla yogurt

Core the apple and place in a small glass baking dish. Fill hole with raisins, walnuts, and cinnamon. Pour orange juice in the bottom of the pan. Cover and bake at 350^0 F until tender. Top with vanilla yogurt. Serves 1.

Sweet Potato Surprise[19]

1 baked sweet potato cut in half lengthwise
2 Tb walnuts
1 Tb honey

1 Tb semi-sweet chocolate chips

Cut open the sweet potato lengthwise. Place walnuts, honey, and chocolate chips on top. Broil 6 inches from heat, until chocolate starts to melt. Serves 1.

Mixed Berry Crisp

2 cups frozen blueberries, blackberries, and/or raspberries
4 Tb healthy butter (flax and butter mixed)
1/2 tsp cinnamon
½ cup whole wheat or spelt flour
¾ cup oats
2 Tb honey

Place frozen berries in a pie pan or 8x8 square pan. Mix 3 tablespoons of butter, cinnamon, flour, oats, and honey until it resembles bread crumbs. Cut up the remaining tablespoon of butter and mix into the berries. Spread the flour/oat mixture evenly on top of the berries. Bake at 375^0 F until the top is browned (approximately 20 minutes). Serve with 1-2 tablespoons of vanilla yogurt or glass of soy, rice, or almond milk. Serves 2.

Peanut Butter Honey Crunch

2 Tb organic peanut butter
1 cup nonfat yogurt
1 Tb sunflower seeds
1 Tb honey

Mix peanut butter with yogurt. Sprinkle sunflower seeds and drizzle honey. Serves 1.

Zucchini or Carrot Bread

This recipe is modified from A Taste of History[20] Zucchini bread.

1 egg
1 medium ripe banana, mashed
1/2 cup honey
1 cup oil
¼ tsp baking powder
2 tsp baking soda
2 cups flour
1 tsp cinnamon or to taste
1 tsp salt
1 tsp vanilla
2 cups grated zucchini or carrots, peeled
1 cup chopped nuts

Mix ingredients in order in a large bowl until well mixed. Grease 1 large loaf pan and fill with batter evenly. Bake one hour at 350°F, or until a wooden pick comes out clean. Cool 15 minutes and remove from pan. Makes 1 loaf.

Dressings, Healthy Fats and Oils

Healthy Cheese/Tofu Spread[21]

3 Tb fresh flax seed oil
7 Tb baker's cheese, cottage cheese, yogurt, or soft tofu
2-3 Tb finely shredded green onions, parsley, grated carrots, green and red bell peppers, chopped tomatoes, and any other fresh vegetables (optional)

Mix thoroughly and refrigerate. Makes ¾ to 1 cup. It tastes great on crackers, bread, or used as a dip for carrots, celery, or apples.

Garlic Hummus

    2 cans chickpeas, rinsed and drained
    1/4 cup water
    2 Tb fresh lemon juice (or lime juice)
    4 cloves to a half head roasted garlic
    Cumin to taste
    Celtic sea salt to taste
    1 Tb sesame tahini (can use more if desired)
    1 Tb good olive oil (can use more if desired)

First, roast your garlic (very important). This recipe will not taste the same if you skip this step. Roasting the garlic gives this hummus a nice mellow, yet rich flavor. To do this, wrap garlic head in foil, then place in 350^0F oven (or toaster oven) for 30 minutes.

Combine all ingredients in food processor or blender and puree until desired smoothness. Add more liquid if desired.

Ginger Dressing[22]

    3 Tb flaxseed oil
    1-2 Tb fresh lemon juice
    1 tsp fresh grated ginger
    1 clove garlic, minced

Whisk together and use as a light dressing over lettuce, grains, vegetables, etc. Refrigerate in an opaque, closed container.

Julie Anne's Tahini Dressing

The recipe is one of my favorite things to drizzle on salads, brown rice, and steamed vegetables. Julie Anne Flynn, a colleague and friend, introduced me to this fabulous recipe.

1 cup vegetable oil
¾ cup apple cider vinegar
½ cup soy sauce
½ cup tahini (sesame seed butter)
2 cloves garlic
½ tsp basil
½ tsp oregano

Mix vinegar and garlic in a blender puree. Add all the rest of the ingredients. Puree 2-3 minutes. Chill and serve.

Chimichurri

Chimichurri is an Argentinean tangy garlic parsley sauce used to top many different meat dishes such as steak, sea bass, chicken, salmon etc. The recipe is adapted from Rebecca Christensen's (Executive Chef of the Blue Vervain Restaurant) recipe. It is full of immune boosting garlic, and thyme and tastes delicious. Parsley is high in vitamin C, vitamin A, and folic acid.

1 cup packed fresh parsley leaves, finely chopped
2 Tb fresh thyme, finely chopped
5 medium garlic cloves, minced
2 Tb water
½ cup extra virgin olive oil
Salt and pepper to taste
¼ cup finely minced red onion
¼ cup red wine vinegar
¼ tsp red pepper flakes

Mix together ingredients by hand and season to taste. Use to top meat or baked tofu dishes.

Tamari Dressing[23]

¼ cup flaxseed oil
2-3 Tb tamari or soy sauce
2-3 Tb apple cider vinegar
1-3 cloves minced garlic
1-2 tsp honey or brown rice syrup (optional)

Whisk together and use as a light dressing over any foods. Refrigerate in an opaque, closed container.

Dill Dressing[24]

1/3 cup minced fresh dill
¼ cup cider vinegar or lemon juice
1-1/2 Tb Dijon mustard
½ tsp honey or rice syrup
½ cup flaxseed oil

Whisk together all ingredients except the flaxseed oil and trickle
that in last until the dressing is thick and smooth. Use over fish,
grains, and vegetables. Refrigerate in an opaque, closed
container.

Healthier Mayonnaise[25]

½ cup flaxseed oil
½ cup oil of your choice (safflower, canola oil, sunflower oil,
    olive oil, etc.)
1 egg
2 Tb lemon juice or vinegar
Dash dry mustard powder
Dash cayenne or ground pepper

Combine egg, lemon juice, mustard, cayenne or pepper with ¼
cup oil mixture in a blender. Blend at a low speed until it begins
to thicken. Immediately add all the remaining oil in a heavy
stream as you continue to blend at low speed. Do not double
recipe or mixing problems may ensue. Refrigerate in an opaque,
closed container. Makes 1-1/2 cups.

Sample Immune Boosting Diet

This sample diet is modified from Chris Cavanaugh's 7 Day Immune Boosting Diet.[26]

Day 1

Breakfast
Immune Boosting Smoothie
Lunch
Cream of Pumpkin Soup

One cup Vegetable Juice
Snacks
1 orange

1 ounce 60-70% dark chocolate
Dinner
Ham Fried Rice
Dessert
Mayan Chocolate Shake

Day 2

Breakfast
Egg Free French Toast

One whole orange or ½ cup orange juice diluted with ½ cup water
Lunch
Beets and Goat Cheese Salad
Snacks
2 cups cubed watermelon or apples (depending on season)

1 ounce raw cashew nuts

Dinner
   Shiitake Chicken
   Steamed ½ acorn squash, sprinkled with 1/8 teaspoon ground
   cinnamon
Dessert
   Mixed Berry Crisp

Day 3

Breakfast
   1 cup Spicy Immune Tea
   1/2 cup nonfat yogurt with 1 tablespoon walnuts and 1/2 cup diced
   papaya
Lunch
   Thai Gazpacho
   Corn chips or sprouted grain/whole wheat pita
Snacks
   Hummus and baby carrots
   1 cup green tea
Dinner
   Lemon Grilled Salmon
Dessert
   Sweet Potato Delight

Day 4

Breakfast
   Immune Support Breakfast
   1 cup green tea
Lunch
   Chicken Pesto Pasta
Snacks

1 cup Mary Bove Immune Tea

½ cup low -fat cottage cheese with ½ cup of fruit or berries

Dinner

Tuna with Mexican Bean Salsa: Season 5 ounces of fresh tuna with salt and pepper. Grill or broil 4 inches from heat for 6-8 minutes. Top with bean salsa.

Dessert

Old-Fashioned Baked Apple

Day 5

Breakfast

Whole grain waffles topped with ½ cup blueberries and 1 tablespoon honey

1 cup green tea

Lunch

Shrimp Salad Pita

Snacks

1 apple dipped in 2 tablespoons nut butter

1 cup Spicy Immune Tea

Dinner

Vegetable Lasagna

Fresh spinach salad with Tahini Dressing

Dessert

Peanut Butter and Honey Crunch

---

[1] Tierra, L. (2000). *A kids herb book*. San Francisco, CA: Robert. R. Reed Publishing.

[2] Bove, Mary. (2001). *An encyclopedia of natural healing for children and infants*. Chicago, IL: Keats.

[3] Tierra, L. (2000). *A kids herb book*. San Francisco, CA: Robert. R. Reed Publishing.

[4] Tierra, L. (2000). *A kids herb book*. San Francisco, CA: Robert. R. Reed Publishing.

[5] Tierra, L. (2000). *A kids herb book*. San Francisco, CA: Robert. R. Reed Publishing.

[6] Tierra, L. (2000). *A kids herb book*. San Francisco, CA: Robert. R. Reed Publishing.

[7] Tierra, L. (2000). *A kids herb book*. San Francisco, CA: Robert. R. Reed Publishing.

[8] *Taste of History Cookbook*. Friends of Hot Springs Public Library Building Fund Raiser.

[9] Cavanaugh, Christopher. (2001) Strengthen Your Immune System. *The Reader's Digest Association*.

[10] Hartung, T. (2000).*Growing 101 Herbs That Heal: Gardening techniques, recipes and remedies*. Pownal, VT: Storey Book Publishing.

[11] Bremzen, AV and Welchman, J. (1995). *Terrific Pacific Cookbook*. New York: Workman Publishing.

[12] Cooking Live. *Sweet Potato Soup*. Retrieved March 15, 2007 from http://www.foodnetwork.com/food/recipes/recipe/0,1977,FOOD_9936_13378,00.html

[13] Cavanaugh, Christopher. (2001) Strengthen Your Immune System. *The Reader's Digest Association*.

[14] Young, Kay. (1993). *Wild Seasons: Gathering and Cooling Wild Plants of the Great Plains*. Lincoln, NE: University of Nebraska Press.

[15] Cavanaugh, Christopher. (2001) Strengthen Your Immune System. *The Reader's Digest Association*.

[16] Cavanaugh, Christopher. (2001) Strengthen Your Immune System. *The Reader's Digest Association.*

[17] Cavanaugh, Christopher. (2001) Strengthen Your Immune System. *The Reader's Digest Association.*

[18] Cavanaugh, Christopher. (2001) Strengthen Your Immune System. *The Reader's Digest Association.*

[19] Cavanaugh, Christopher. (2001) Strengthen Your Immune System. *The Reader's Digest Association..*

[20] *Taste of History Cookbook.* Friends of Hot Springs Public Library Building Fund Raiser.

[21] Balch, Phyllis and James. (2000). *Prescriptions for Nutritional Healing,* (3rd ed.). New York: Avery.

[22] Balch, Phyllis and James. (2000). *Prescriptions for Nutritional Healing,* (3rd ed.). New York: Avery.

[23] Balch, Phyllis and James. (2000). *Prescriptions for Nutritional Healing,* (3rd ed.). New York: Avery.

[24] Balch, Phyllis and James. (2000). *Prescriptions for Nutritional Healing,* (3rd ed.). New York: Avery.

[25] Balch, Phyllis and James. (2000). *Prescriptions for Nutritional Healing,* (3rd ed.). New York: Avery.

[26] Cavanaugh, Christopher. (2001) Strengthen Your Immune System. *The Reader's Digest Association.*

Glossary

Adaptogen: Acts to aid the body in coping with and counteracting the effects of stress.

Anticatarrhal: Eliminates or decreases the formation of mucus in the sinus area, throat, and lungs.

Antimicrobial: Kills a variety of bacteria and viruses.

Antiseptic: Prevents infection by inhibiting the growth of micro-organisms on living tissue.

Antitussive: Inhibits coughing.

Carminative: Expels gas from the stomach and intestines and thus helps to relieve colic, and gas pains, and relaxes the stomach.

Decoction: A way to prepare tea from the roots or seeds or dried berries of a plant. The roots and seeds are simmered in hot water for 15 minutes, strained, and then taken as a tea.

Diaphoretic: Promotes sweating when used as a hot tea. Diaphoretics can bring down a fever by promoting sweating.

Expectorant: Aids in expelling mucus from the lungs and throat.

Glycerite: A way to preserve, concentrate, and sweeten herbs. Instead of using grain alcohol like tinctures do, in glycerites, a sweet alcohol is used to extract and preserve key nutrients. Glycerites are most often used for children.

Infusion: A way to prepare tea using the flowers, leaves, and stems of a plant. Boiled water is poured over the herbs and steeped, covered, with a lid for 15 minutes, strained, and then taken as a tea.

Immunomodulator: Acts to restore, enhance, and improve the body's immune function and response.

Immune Stimulating: Acts by stimulating different parts of the immune system.

Mucolytic: Breaks up and resolves mucus.

Nervine: Soothes and relieves tension without sedation. It may stimulate or relax the body.

Syrup: A way to take herbs by mixing an infusion, decoction, or tincture with honey or sugar. Syrups are used most often in cough syrups to soothe the throat and in herbal preparations for children over 1 year old. It is best to refrigerate after mixing.

Tincture: An herbal preparation using water and alcohol to extract key nutrients of herbs concentrate them and preserve their effectiveness.

Tonic: Improves tone by improving tissue nutrition. Tonics invigorate, restore the system, and promotes optimal tissue tone. Tonics can be whole body tonics or specific to a particular organ system.

Research

Sugar and the Immune System

Differential effects of honey, sucrose, and fructose on blood sugar levels. (1991). Shambaugh P, Worthington V, Herbert JH. Journal of Manipulative and physiological therapeutics. Jan;14(1):91-2.

It is now recognized that dietary carbohydrate components influence the prevalence and severity of common degenerative diseases such as dental problems, diabetes, heart disease, and obesity. Fructose and sucrose have been evaluated and compared to glucose using glucose tolerance tests, but few such comparisons have been performed for a "natural" sugar source such as honey. In this study, 33 upper trimester chiropractic students volunteered for oral glucose tolerance testing comparing sucrose, fructose, and honey during successive weeks. A 75-gm carbohydrate load in 250 ml of water was ingested and blood sugar readings were taken at 0, 30, 60, 90, 120 and 240 minutes. Fructose showed minimal changes in blood sugar levels, consistent with other studies. Sucrose gave higher blood sugar readings than honey at every measurement, producing significantly (p less than .05) greater glucose intolerance. Honey provided the fewest subjective symptoms of discomfort. Given that honey has a gentler effect on blood sugar levels on a per gram basis, and tastes sweeter than sucrose so that fewer grams would be consumed, it would seem prudent to recommend honey over sucrose.

Sucrose, neutrophilic phagocytosis and resistance to disease. (1976). Ringsdorf WM Jr, Cheraskin E, Ramsay RR Jr.. Dentistry Survey.Dec;52(12):46-8.

Anti-Inflammatory and Immunomodulatory Activities of Stevioside and Its Metabolite Steviol on THP-1 Cells. (2006). Boonkaewwan C, Toskulkao C, Vongsakul M. Journal of agriculture and food chemistry. Feb 8;54(3):785-9.

Stevioside, a natural noncaloric sweetener isolated from Stevia rebaudiana Bertoni, possesses anti-inflammatory and antitumor promoting properties; however, no information is available to explain its activity. The anti-inflammatory and immunomodulatory activities of stevioside and its metabolite, steviol, were studied. Stevioside at 1 mM significantly suppressed lipopolysaccharide (LPS)-induced release of TNF-alpha and IL-1beta and slightly suppressed nitric oxide release in THP-1 cells without exerting any direct toxic effect, whereas steviol at 100 microM did not. This study suggested that stevioside attenuates synthesis of inflammatory mediators in LPS-stimulated THP-1 cells by interfering with the IKKbeta and NF-kappaB signaling pathway, and stevioside-induced TNF-alpha secretion is partially mediated through TLR4.

Digestive System and Immune Function

Review article: mechanisms of initiation and perpetuation of gut inflammation by stress. Hart, A and Kamm, MA. (2002) Alimentary Pharmacology and Therapeutics. Dec;16(12):2017-28.

Stress can alter intestinal physiological function. Stress can increase gut permeability, increase ion secretion by a mechanism involving neural stimulation or mast cells, increase mucin release, and deplete goblet cells. Stress causes parasympathetic activation via a mechanism involving corticotropin releasing factor, ultimately affecting mucosal mast cells. Stress also results in increased bacterial adherence and decreased luminal lactobacilli. As a result of all these changes, luminal antigens may gain access to the epithelium, causing inflammation.

Resident bacterial flora and immune system. Biancone, L et al. (2002). Digestive and Liver Disease. 2002 Sep;34 Suppl 2:S37-43.

The intestinal mucosa represents a considerable proportion of the human immune system. Dysregulation of the mucosal immune response can switch a "controlled" toward an "uncontrolled" intestinal inflammation. A key role in the maintenance of an adequate balance between antigenic stimulation and host immune response is played by the immunoregulatory molecules released by activated immunocytes in the human gut. The role of the host immune system in the maintenance of an adequate balance between luminal antigens, including the resident bacterial flora and host immune response, is strongly supported by animal models of uncontrolled intestinal inflammation.

The resident bacterial flora seems to play a major role in the development of animal models of "uncontrolled" intestinal inflammation through immune molecules. Probiotics, defined as living micro-organisms, when taken in appropriate amounts, improve the health status of the digestive system.

Sleep and The Immune System

Poor sleep the night before an experimental stressor predicts reduced NK cell mobilization and slowed recovery in healthy women. (2006). Wright, CE et al. Brain, behavior, and immunity. Oct 5; [Epub ahead of print]

Alterations in immune function following poor sleep (defined by duration and disruption) may be linked to ill health. Not yet investigated are the possible effects on stress-induced mobilization of lymphocytes. As natural killer (NK) cells are particularly responsive to acute stress, the present study examined whether sleep period duration and percentage of time awake after sleep onset (WASO) the night before a laboratory stressor would predict reduced NK cell mobilization.

Sleep was monitored in 39 healthy women. NK cell peripheral blood numbers were determined at baseline (post-20minutes rest), 4 minutes into a Stroop task, immediately post-task and 30minutes after task completion. Participants with high WASO had significantly less NK cell mobilization to the stressor and failed to return to baseline levels after 30 minutes compared to women with low WASO.

No effects were found for sleep period duration. Findings raise the possibility that inadequate NK cell mobilization to, and poor recovery from, acute stress may be one pathway by which sleep could impact health.

Partial night sleep deprivation reduces natural killer and cellular immune responses in humans. (1996). Irwin, M et al. The FASEB journal. Apr;10(5):643-53

Prolonged and severe sleep deprivation is associated with alterations of natural and cellular immune function. The effects of early-night partial sleep deprivation on circulating numbers of white blood cells, natural killer (NK) cell number and cytotoxicity, lymphokine-activated killer (LAK) cell number and activity, and stimulated interleukin-2 (IL-2) production were studied in 42 medically and psychiatrically healthy male volunteers.

After a night of sleep deprivation between 10 P.M. and 3 A.M., a reduction of natural immune responses as measured by NK cell activity, and LAK activity was found. In addition, IL-2 production was suppressed after sleep deprivation due to changes in both adherent and nonadherent cell populations. After a night of recovery sleep, NK activity returned to baseline levels and but IL-2 production remained suppressed. These data implicate sleep in the modulation of immunity and demonstrate that even a modest disturbance of sleep produces a reduction of natural immune responses and T cell cytokine production. **Shift of monocyte function toward cellular immunity during sleep.(2006). Lange, T et al. Archives of Internal Medicine. Sep 18;166(16):1695-700.**

Sleep is considered to strengthen immune defense. We hypothesized that sleep achieves this effect by shifting the balance between types 1 and 2 cytokine activity toward increased type 1 activity, thereby supporting adaptive cellular immune responses. Monocyte-derived type 1 (interleukin 12 [IL-12]) and type 2 (IL-10) cytokines were analyzed in 11 healthy subjects during a regular sleep-wake cycle and 24 hours of wakefulness. The results showed that sleep increased the number of IL-12-producing monocytes and concurrently decreased the number of IL-10-producing monocytes, thereby inducing clear rhythms in these cells, with maximum numbers at 2:20 and 11:30 am, respectively. The rhythms were completely absent during continuous wakefulness. Other studies suggest that high prolactin and low cortisol levels are factors contributing to the shift in the IL-12/IL-10 ratio toward increased IL-12 activity during sleep.

In conclusion, IL-12 and IL-10 play a critical role between antigen-presenting cells and lymphocytes. By preferentially supporting type 1 IL-12 activity, sleep induces a 24-hour oscillation between type 1 and 2 cytokines and, in this way, acts to globally increase the efficacy of adaptive immune responses. Improving sleep represents a therapeutic option to enhance the success of vaccinations and in the treatment of atopic dermatitis, auto immune diseases and human immunodeficiency virus infection) that are characterized by type 2 cytokine over activity.

Toxins and the Immune System

Disturbance of human immunohomeostasis by environmental pollution and alcohol consumption. (2006). Kazbariene, B, Krikstaponiene, A and Monceviciute-Eringiene, E. Acta microbiologica et immunologica Hungarica Jun;53(2):209-18.

Environmental pollution and consumption of alcohol evoke various immunomodulation's promoting the progress of different pathologies. The purpose of this study was to evaluate the influence of alcohol consumption intensity on the immune system functions of humans living in ecologically different regions, i.e. in a district polluted with industrial siftings (Trakai, n = 270) and in a relatively clean district (Sirvintos, n = 250). In the Trakai cohort 96% and in Sirvintos group 89% of persons consumed alcohol. With regard to alcohol consumption habits the white blood cell numbers were investigated in the following four groups: abstinents, light alcohol users, moderate alcohol users and alcohol abusers. We determined the compensatory mechanisms of immune system functions of moderate alcohol users and alcohol abusers in comparison with abstinents in the relatively clean Sirvintos district. In the Trakai district polluted with industrial siftings such compensatory reactions were not found. Thus, damage to the immune system functions is not only an endogenous risk factor for many diseases, but also an indicator of organism injury. This investigation stated, that immunity disturbance in humans depends on alcohol consumption intensity and place of residence.

Daily moderate amounts of red wine or alcohol have no effect on the immune system of healthy men. (2004). Watzl, B. et al. European Journal of Clinical Nutrition. Jan;58(1):40-5.

This study investigated whether the daily intake of red wine (RW) at a dose which inversely correlates with cardiovascular disease (CVD) risk modulates immune functions in healthy men. A total of 24 healthy males with moderate alcohol consumption patterns were recruited and all completed the study. Participants consumed approximately 16 oz of either red wine, dealcoholized red wine, grape juice or 12% alcoholic beverage.

Immune parameters were measured a few weeks before consumption, during consumption and after consumption. The results showed that consumption of a moderate volume of alcohol with RW and with a 12% ETOH dilution had no effect on immune functions in healthy males. Daily moderate consumption of alcohol and of RW for 2 weeks at doses which inversely correlate with CVD risk has no adverse effects on human immune cell functions. Polyphenol-rich beverages such as RGJ and DRW further do not suppress immune responses in healthy men.

Immunosuppression in the mouse induced by long-term exposure to cigarette smoke.(1978). Holt PG, Keast D, Mackenzie JS. American journal of pathology. Jan;90(1):281-4.

Effects of cigarette smoke on immune response: chronic exposure to cigarette smoke impairs antigen-mediated signaling in T cells and depletes IP3-sensitive Ca(2+) stores.(2000). Kalra R, Singh SP, Savage SM, Finch GL, Sopori ML. Journal of pharmacology and experimental therapeutics.Apr;293(1):166-71.

Chronic exposure of mice and rats to cigarette smoke affects T-cell responsiveness that may account for the decreased T-cell proliferative and T-dependent antibody responses in humans and animals exposed to cigarette smoke. Our laboratory has shown that chronic exposure of rats to nicotine inhibits the antibody-forming cell response, impairs the antigen-mediated signaling in T cells, and induces T cell energy. To determine the mechanism of cigarette smoke-induced immunosuppression and to compare it with chronic nicotine exposure, rats were exposed to diluted, mainstream cigarette smoke for up to 30 months or to nicotine for 4 weeks, and evaluated for immunological function in vivo and in vitro. This article presents evidence suggesting that T cells from long-term cigarette smoke-exposed rats exhibit decreased antigen-mediated proliferation and constitutive activation of protein tyrosine kinase and phospholipase C-gamma1 activities. Moreover, spleen cells from smoke-exposed and nicotine-treated animals have depleted inositol-1, 4,5-trisphosphate-sensitive Ca(2+) stores and a decreased ability to raise intracellular Ca(2+) levels in response to T cell antigen receptor ligation. These results suggest that chronic smoking causes T cell death. Moreover, nicotine may account for or contribute to the immunosuppressive properties of cigarette smoke.

Stress and The Immune System

A single social defeat transiently suppresses the anti-viral immune response in mice. (1999). De Groot, J et al. Journal of neruoimmunology. Mar 1;95(1-2):143-51.

Most of the studies dealing with effects of stress on anti-viral immunity have been carried out with stressors that are of long duration and that bear little relationship to the nature of the species. In this paper, we investigated the effect of a stressor mimicking real-life situations more closely, being social defeat of male mice, on anti-viral immunity.

A single social defeat was applied at 3 or 6 days after inoculation with pseudorabies virus, a herpes virus. It appeared that lymph node cellularity, virus specific IL-2 and IFN-gamma production and lymphocyte proliferation were suppressed at 1 day after defeat, but these parameters restored to control values quickly thereafter. We conclude that the stress of a single social defeat evokes a transient immune suppression, which might have consequences if a pathogenic or lethal virus is involved.

**Immunological responses to social stress: dependence
on social environment and coping abilities.** (1993).
Bohus, B, Koolhass, JM, Heijnen, CJ and de Boer,O.
Neuropsychobiology. 28(1-2):95-9.

Social interactions as a consequence of the social
position represent stressful conditions for the individual.
Manipulation of social conditions or forming long-term
social hierarchies by colony aggregation allow to
investigate the regulation of immune defense mechanisms
under seminatural circumstances. Social stimulation
without aggressive interactions increases the relative
number of T-helper cells, whereas defeat leads to an
increase in the T-suppressor/cytotoxic subpopulation. The
data suggest multiple and differential effects of social stress
on immune system functioning in the rat. Individual
characteristics of the coping with stress, the social
environment, and the immune indices under investigation
determine the magnitude and direction of the changes in
immune functioning.

**Stress, cancer and immunity. New developments in
biopsychosocial and psychoneuroimmunologic research.
(1991). Baltrusch HJ, Stangel W, Titze I. Acta
neurologica. Aug;13(4):315-27.**

Research in biobehavioral oncology focuses on stress as
one dispositional factor in the multifactorial origin and in
the clinical progression of cancer Recently, behavioral
oncologists have similarly attempted at conceptualizing a
"Type C" or biopsychosocial cancer risk pattern, as they
have noted the denial and suppression of emotions, in

particular anger. Other features of this pattern are "pathological niceness", avoidance of conflicts, exaggerated social desirability, harmonizing behavior, over-compliance, over-patience, as well as high rationality and a rigid control of emotional expression ("anti-emotionality"). This pattern, usually concealed behind a facade of pleasantness, appears to be effective as long as environmental and psychological homeostasis is maintained, but collapses in the course of time under the impact of accumulated strains and stressors.

As a prominent feature of this particular coping style, excessive denial, avoidance, suppression and repression of emotions and own basic needs appears to weaken the organism's natural resistance to carcinogenic influences. This may mean that the excessive use of denial and suppression/repression has important psychophysiologic effects linked to tumor biology and host-defense.

Recent studies reveal that psychosocial stressors which are met by inadequate and repressive coping styles are associated with changes in immunocompetence, including both humoral and cell-mediated immunity. Relationships between different immune parameters (natural killer cell activity, lymphocytes, serotonin uptake, mean platelet volume) and mood states, psychological coping styles and personality variables are outlined.

Psychoneuroendocrine immunology: perception of stress can alter body temperature and natural killer cell activity. (1998). Hiramoto RN, Solvason HB, Hsueh CM, Rogers CF, Demissie S, Hiramoto NS, Gauthier DK, Lorden JF, Ghanta VK. International journal of neruoscience. 98(1-2):95-129.

Psychoimmunology has been credited with using the mind as a way to alter immunity. The problem with this concept is that many of the current psychoimmunology techniques in use are aimed at alleviating stress effects on the immune system rather than at direct augmentation of immunity by the brain. Studies in animals provide a model that permits us to approach the difficulties associated with gaining an understanding of the CNS-immune system connection. We emphasize conditioning as a regimen and an acceptable way to train the brain to remember an output pathway to raise immunity. We propose that a specific drug or perception (mild stress, represented by rotation, total body heating or handling) could substitute and kindle the same output pathway without the need for conditioning. If this view is correct, then instead of using conditioning, it may be possible to use an antigen to activate desired immune cells, and substitute a drug or an external environmental sensory stimulus (perception) to energize the output pathway to these cells.

Alternatively, monitoring alterations of body temperature in response to a drug or perception might allow us to follow how effectively the brain is performing in altering immunity. Studies with animals suggest that there are alternative ways to use the mind to raise natural or acquired immunity in man.

Emotions and the Immune System

The immune system and happiness. (2006). Barak, Y. Autoimmune Review. Oct;5(8):523-7. Epub 2006 Mar 21.

The complex interactions between the immune system and the central nervous system have been studied extensively in schizophrenia and depression. On the other hand, effects of positive human emotions, especially happiness, on physiological parameters and immunity have received very little attention. Emotions are intimately involved in the initiation or progression of cancer, HIV, cardiovascular disease, and autoimmune disorders. The specific physiological responses induced by pleasant stimuli were recently investigated with the immune and endocrine systems being monitored when pleasant stimuli such as odors and emotional pictures were presented to subjects.

The results revealed that an increase in secretory immunoglobulin A and a decrease in salivary cortisol were induced by pleasant emotions. There is data to support the hypothesis that individuals characterized by a more negative affective style poorly recruit their immune response and may be at risk for illness more so than those with a positive affective style. Future research is needed to expand our knowledge of the physiological and immune interactions of positive emotional states and their beneficial effects on health.

Exercise and the Immune System

The effects of long-term endurance training on the immune and endocrine systems of elderly men: the role of cytokines and anabolic hormones. Aria, MH, Duarte, AJ, and Natale, VM. (2006). *Immune Ageing.* **Aug 25;3:9.**

This study examined the immune and endocrine system of elderly men that exercised and those that did not. The elderly runners showed a significantly higher T cell proliferative response and IL-2 production than sedentary elderly controls. IL-2 production was similar to that in young adults. Their serum IL-6 levels were significantly lower than their sedentary peers. They also showed significantly lower IL-3 production in comparison to sedentary elderly subjects but similar to the young. Anabolic hormone levels did not differ between elderly groups and no clear correlation was found between hormones and cytokine levels. Long-term endurance training has the potential to decelerate the age-related decline in immune function but not the deterioration in endocrine function.

Effects of 6 months of moderate aerobic exercise training on immune function in the elderly. Woods, JA et al.(1999). *Mechanism of Ageing Dev.* **Jun 1;109(1):1-19.**

Previously sedentary elderly (age= 65 +/- 0.8 years) subjects were randomly assigned to supervised 3 time/week exercise intervention group (EXC, n = 14) or flexibility/toning control group (FT-CON, n = 15). Fasting resting blood samples were drawn prior to and after the 6 month intervention. Immune results revealed that, in general, changes in immune function in response to 6 months of exercise training at an average intensity of 52% heart rate reserve (HRR) were similar when compared to FT-CON who exercised at approximately 21% HRR. There were no intervention-induced changes in total white blood cell, neutrophil, lymphocyte, monocyte, eosinophil, or basophil blood counts. Furthermore, the percentage and number of CD3+, CD4+ and CD8+ T cells in the blood remained unchanged. There was a tendency for the percentage and number of CD4+ and CD8+ naive cells (CD45RA+) to increase and for CD4+ memory cells (CD45RO+) to decrease post-intervention, especially in FT-CON.

Both groups exhibited a small intervention-induced increase in the T-cell proliferative response to mitogenic stimulation: the percentage change of which was higher in the EXC group. Unstimulated NK cell cytolysis versus K562 cells tended to increase ($P < 0.1$) in the EXC group with little change in FT-CON. We conclude that 6 months of supervised exercise training can lead to nominal increases in some measures of immune function, while not affecting others, in previously sedentary elderly.

**Physical activity and immune function in elderly women.
Nieman, DC et al. (1993).** *Medical Science Sports
Exercise.* **Jul;25(7):823-31.**

The relationship between cardio-respiratory exercise,
immune function, and upper respiratory tract infection
(URTI) was studied in elderly women utilizing a
randomized controlled experimental design with a follow-
up of 12 wk. Thirty-two sedentary, elderly Caucasian
women, 67-85 yr. of age, who met specific selection
criteria, were randomized to either a walking or callisthenic
group; 30 completed the study. Twelve highly conditioned
elderly women, 65-84 yr. of age, who were active in
endurance competitions, were recruited at baseline for
cross-sectional comparisons.

Intervention groups exercised 30-40 minutes, 5 days a
wk-1, for 12 wk., with the walking group training at 60%
heart rate reserve and the callisthenic group engaging in
mild range-of-motion and flexibility movements that kept
their heart rates close to resting levels. At baseline, the
highly conditioned subjects exhibited superior NK cell
function, despite no differences in circulating levels of
lymphocyte subpopulations. Twelve weeks of moderate
cardio-respiratory exercise did not result in any
improvement in NK cell activity or T cell function.
Incidence of URTI was lowest in the highly conditioned
group and highest in the callisthenic control group during
the 12-wk study, with the walkers in an intermediate
position (chi-square = 6.36, P = 0.042). In conclusion, the
highly conditioned elderly women in this study had

superior NK and T cell function when compared with their sedentary counterparts.

Nutrition and Immune System

Garlic and aging: new insights into an old remedy. (2003). Rahman, K. Ageing research reviews. Jan;2(1):39-56.

There has been an impressive gain in individual life expectancy with parallel increases in age-related chronic diseases of the cardiovascular, brain and immune systems. These can cause loss of autonomy, dependence and high social costs for individuals and society. It is now accepted that aging and age-related diseases are in part caused by free radical reactions. The arrest of aging and stimulation of rejuvenation of the human body is also being sought. Over the last 20 years the use of herbs and natural products has gained popularity and these are being consumed backed by epidemiological evidence. One such herb is garlic, which has been used throughout the history of civilization for treating a wide variety of ailments associated with aging.

The role of garlic in preventing age-related diseases has been investigated extensively over the last 10-15 years. Garlic has strong antioxidant properties and it has been suggested that garlic can prevent cardiovascular disease, inhibit platelet aggregation, thrombus formation, prevent cancer, diseases associated with cerebral aging, arthritis, cataract formation, and rejuvenate skin, improve blood circulation and energy levels. This review provides an insight in to garlic's antioxidant properties and presents evidence that it may either prevent or delay chronic diseases associated with aging.

Garlic extracts stimulate proliferation of rat lymphocytes in vitro by increasing IL-2 and IL-4 production. (2000). Colic, M and Savic, M. Immunopharmacology and immunotoxicology. Feb;22(1):163-81.

Garlic components are known to modulate certain immune functions. However, mechanisms of their action are not sufficiently elucidated. This study was, therefore, undertaken to examine the effects of aqueous and ethanolic extracts prepared from a garlic powder sample on proliferation of rat spleen lymphocytes in culture. The results suggest that the potentiating effect of garlic extracts on lymphocyte proliferation in vitro differs depending on specific stimulators of cell proliferation and probably on the type of responding cells.

Hormones and the Immune System

A regulatory role of prolactin, growth hormone, and corticosteroids for human T-cell production of cytokines. (2004) Dimitrov, S, Lange, T, Fehm, HL, Born, J. Brain, behavior, and immunity. Jul;18(4):368-74

The release of the pituitary hormones, prolactin and growth hormone (GH), and of adrenal corticosteroids is subject to a profound regulation by sleep. In addition these hormones are known to be involved in the regulation of the immune response. Here, we examined their role for in vitro production of T-cell cytokines. Specifically, we hypothesized that increased concentrations of prolactin and GH as well as a decrease in cortisol, i.e., hormonal changes characterizing early nocturnal sleep, could be responsible for a shift towards T helper 1 (Th1) cytokines during this time. Whole blood was sampled from 15 healthy humans in the morning after regular sleep were studied. Results suggest that enhanced prolactin and GH concentrations as well as low cortisol levels during early nocturnal sleep synergistically act to enhance Th1 cytokine activity.

Effect of gender and sex hormones on immune responses following shock. (2000). Angele, MK, Schwacha, MG, Ayala, A, Chaudry, IH. Shock. Aug;14(2):81-90.

Several clinical and experimental studies show a gender difference of the immune and organ responsiveness in the susceptibility to and morbidity from shock, trauma, and sepsis. In this respect, cell-mediated immune responses are depressed in males after trauma-hemorrhage, whereas they are unchanged or enhanced in females. Sex hormones contribute to this gender-specific immune response after adverse circulatory conditions. Specifically, studies indicate that androgens are responsible for the immunodepression after trauma-hemorrhage in males. In contrast, female sex steroids seem to exhibit immunoprotective properties after trauma and severe blood loss, because administration of estrogen prevents the androgen-induced immunodepression in castrated male mice.

Nonetheless, the precise underlying mechanisms for these immunomodulatory effects of sex steroids after shock remain unknown. Although testosterone depletion, testosterone receptor antagonism, or estrogen treatment has been shown to prevent the depression of immune functions after trauma-hemorrhage, it remains to be established whether differences in the testosterone-estradiol ratio are responsible for the immune dysfunction. Furthermore, sex hormone receptors have been identified on various immune cells, suggesting direct effects.

Effects of testosterone, 17beta-estradiol, and downstream estrogens on cytokine secretion from human leukocytes in the presence and absence of cortisol. (2006). Janele, D. et al. Annals of the New York Academy of Sciences. Jun;1069:168-82

Estrogens at physiological concentrations are thought to play an immune-stimulating role, whereas androgens have an anti-inflammatory impact. However, their role on cytokine secretion in the presence or absence of cortisol has not been investigated. In this study on peripheral blood leukocytes of healthy male subjects, we scrutinized the influence of prior sex hormones (for 24 h) with and without later addition of cortisol (for another 24 h) on stimulated secretion of TNF, IL-2, IL-4, IL-6, IL-10, and interferon-gamma (IFN-gamma).

At physiological concentrations, E2 and a combination of downstream estrogens stabilized or increased immune stimuli-induced TNF secretion. These effects are dependent on the presence of physiological concentrations of cortisol. This study underlines the proinflammatory role of E2, which is probably dependent on conversion to a proinflammatory cocktail of downstream estrogens and the presence of cortisol.

Immunomodulating Herbs

Modulation of cytokine expression by traditional medicines: a review of herbal immunomodulators. Spellman, K et al. Altern Med Rev. 2006 Jun;11(2):128-50.

A class of herbal medicines, known as immunomodulators, alters the activity of immune function through the dynamic regulation of informational molecules such as cytokines. This may offer an explanation of the effects of herbs on the immune system and other tissues. Many medicinal plant extracts had effects on at least one cytokine. The most frequently studied cytokines were IL-1, IL-6, TNF, and IFN. Acalypha wilkesiana, Acanthopanax gracilistylus, Allium sativum, Ananus comosus, Cissampelos sympodialis, Coriolus versicolor, Curcuma longa, Echinacea purpurea, Grifola frondosa, Harpagophytum procumbens, Panax ginseng, Polygala tenuifolia, Poria cocos, Silybum marianum, Smilax glabra, Tinospora cordifolia, Uncaria tomentosa, and Withania somnifera demonstrate modulation of multiple cytokines. The in vitro and in vivo research demonstrates that the reviewed botanical medicines modulate the secretion of multiple cytokines. The reported therapeutic success of these plants by traditional cultures and modern clinicians may be partially due to their effects on cytokines. Phytotherapy offers a potential therapeutic modality for the treatment of many differing conditions involving cytokines. Given the cytokine modulation, further study of these herbs on cytokine-related diseases such as autoimmune conditions and chronic degenerative processes is warranted.

Adaptogenic activity of Withania somnifera: an experimental study using a rat model of chronic stress. Bhattacharya, SK and Muruganandam, AV (2003). *Pharmacol Biochem Behav.* Jun;75(3):547-55.

The adaptogenic activity of a standardized extract of Ashwagandha roots was investigated against a rat model of chronic stress. The chronic stress induced significant hyperglycemia, glucose intolerance, increase in plasma corticosteroid levels, gastric ulcerations, male sexual dysfunction, cognitive deficits, immunosuppression and mental depression. Ashwagandha significantly decreased the stress induced changes confirming the clinical use of the plant in Ayurveda.

Antimicrobial properties of a non-toxic glycoprotein from Withania somnifera (Ashwagandha)
Girish, LS et al. (2006) *J Basic Microbiol.*46(5):365-74.

A protein designated WSG (Withania somnifera glycoprotein) demonstrated potent antimicrobial activity against the pathogenic fungi and bacteria tested. Antifungal effect has been demonstrated in that WSG exerts a fungistastic effect by inhibiting spore germination and hyphal growth in the tested fungi. WSG showed potent antifungal activity against Aspergillus flavus, Fusarium oxysporum, F. verticilloides and anti-bacterial activity against Clyibacter michiganensis.

Anxiolytic-antidepressant activity of Withania somnifera glycowithanolides: an experimental study. Bhattacharya, SK et. al.(2000).*Phytomedicine.* Dec:7(6): 463-9.

This study compared bioactive glycowithanolides (WSG), isolated from Ashwagandha roots, in rats to the benzodiazepine lorazepam for anxiolytic studies, and by the tricyclic anti-depressant, imipramine, for the antidepressant investigations. Ashwagandha performed equally to the lorazepam group and both decreased a marker of clinical anxiety in the rat brain. WSG also exhibited an antidepressant effect, comparable with that induced by imipramine, in the forced swim-induced 'behavioral despair' and 'learned helplessness' tests.

Efficacy of an extract of North American ginseng containing poly-furanosyl-pyranosyl-saccharides for preventing upper respiratory tract infections: a randomized controlled trial. Predy, GN. (2005). CMAJ. Oct 25; 173(9):1043-8.

In a randomized, double-blind, placebo-controlled study, North American Ginseng was given to people for 4 months. The results showed that subjects who experienced two or more colds during the 4-month period was 50% less in the ginseng group than in the placebo group and the total number of days cold symptoms were 5-6 days shorter for the ginseng group than the placebo group. In summary, American ginseng reduced the mean number of colds per person, the proportion of subjects who experienced 2 or more colds, the severity of symptoms and the number of days cold symptoms were reported.

Peripheral blood mononuclear cell production of TNF-alpha in response to North American ginseng stimulation. Zhou, DL. And Kitts, DD. (2002). Canadian Journal of Physiology and Pharmacology. Oct;80(10):1030-3.

North American ginseng (Panax quinquifolius) root extract (NAGE) with known ginsenosides composition was examined for its ability to stimulate tumor necrosis factor alpha (TNF-alpha) production in human peripheral blood mononuclear cells. The stimulation of TNF-alpha production was confirmed by TNF-alpha mRNA gene expression. These interesting results show the immunostimulating activity of NAGE components in reference to TNF-alpha production. This observation requires further investigation with more subjects to determine the affinity of ginseng in stimulating the human immune system.

Antimicrobial and antiplasmid activities of essential oils. Schelz, Z, Molnar, J and Hohmann, J. (2006). Fitotherapia. Jun;77(4):279-85. Epub 2006 May 11.

The antimicrobial and antiplasmid activities of essential oils (orange oil, eucalyptus oil, fennel oil, geranium oil, juniper oil, peppermint) oil, rosemary oil, purified turpentine effects of American ginseng (Panax quinquifolius) were studied at the onset of the influenza season. A total of 323 subjects 18-65 years of age with a history of at least 2 colds in the previous year were recruited from the general population in Edmonton, Alberta. The participants were instructed to take 2 capsules per day of either the North American ginseng extract or a placebo for a period of 4 months. The mean number of colds per person was lower in the ginseng group than in the placebo group 68% versus 93%. The proportion of subjects with 2 oil, thyme oil, Australian tea tree oil) and of menthol, the main component of peppermint oil, were investigated. The antimicrobial activities were determined on the Gram (+) Staphylococcus epidermidis and the Gram (-) Escherichia coli and on two yeast Saccharomyces cerevisiae.

The antiplasmid activities were investigated on E. coli bacterial strain. Each of the oils exhibited antimicrobial activity and three of them antiplasmid action. The interaction of peppermint oil and menthol with the antibiotics was studied on the same bacterial strain with the checkerboard method. Peppermint oil and menthol displayed increased the anti-bacterial activity of oxytetracycline, an antibiotic.

Ginseng and Salviae herbs play a role as immune activators and modulate immune responses during influenza virus infection. (2006). Quan, FS et al. Vaccine. Aug 10; [Epub ahead of print]

Asian ginseng and sage were studied regarding their effects on early immune responses during influenza virus infection in a mouse model. Intranasal co-administration with inactivated influenza virus A (PR8) and ginseng or sage extract increased the levels of influenza virus specific antibodies and neutralizing activities compared to immunization with PR8 alone, and provided protective immunity. Sage) co-administration significantly enhanced IFN-gamma and IL-2 cytokine producing splenocytes while ginseng induced high levels of IL-4 and IL-5 cytokine producing cells after challenge infection. Sage and ginseng also modulated the immune response so that a proinflammatory cytokine highly elevated in the lungs was not produced protecting against immune mediated damage to the lungs during influenza. These mice also showed significant enhancement of influenza virus specific IgA antibody in lungs after challenge virus infection.

Therefore, these results indicate that both ginseng and sage play a role as mucosal adjuvants against influenza virus as well as immuno-modulators during influenza virus infection.

Echinacea purpurea stimulates cellular immunity and anti-bacterial defense independently of the strain of mice. Bany, J. et al. (2003). Pol J vet Sci. 6(3 Suppl):3-5.

One of the major functions of the immune system is anti-bacterial defense mediated among others by non-specific immunity (macrophages, granulocytes). Echinacea purpurea extracts are widely used in prophylaxis and therapy of various infections, mainly the respiratory tract, in animals and humans. The aim of this work was to evaluate the effect of prophylactic use of Echinacea purpurea extract on the development of Pseudomonas aeruginosa infection in various strains of mice and on some parameters of non-specific and also specific cellular immunity.

Mice expressed various, depending on the strain used, susceptibility to infection. Echinacea feeding resulted in diminishing of bacteria number in livers of susceptible strains as well as the relative resistant strain of mice. Echinacea feeding of the second relative resistant strain resulted in stimulation of granulocytes chemiluminescent and lymphocytes proliferative response.

Antioxidant and immuno-enhancing effects of Echinacea purpurea. Mishima, S et al. Biol Pharm Bull. 2004 Jul;27(7):1004-9.

We studied the protective effects of Echinacea purpurea against radiation by evaluating changes in the peripheral blood cell count and peripheral blood antioxidant activity. E. purpurea administration had a suppressive effect on radiation-induced leukopenia, especially on lymphocytes and monocytes, and resulted in a faster recovery of blood cell counts. Mouse peripheral blood antioxidant activity was increased by E. purpurea, and a relationship between the suppressive effect on radiation-induced leukopenia and the antioxidant effect was suggested. The effects of immune activation by E. purpurea were investigated by measuring total immunoglobulin (IgG, IgM). E. purpurea activates macrophages to stimulate IFN-gamma production in association with the secondary activation of T lymphocytes, resulting in a decrease in IgG and IgM production.

Cytokines released from macrophages in mouse peripheral blood after E. purpurea administration activated helper T cells to proliferate. We think that CD 4 and CD 8 subsets were more immunologically enhanced by E. purpurea than helper T cells and suppressor T cell these results reflect activation. In addition, we think that these results reflect cell-mediated immune responses.

A new extract of the plant Calendula officinalis produces a dual in vitro effect: cytotoxic anti-tumor activity and lymphocyte activation. Jimenez-Medina, E et al. (2006). BMC Cancer. May 5;6:119.

Prior studies of different Calendula extracts have shown anti-inflammatory, anti-viral, and anti-genotoxic properties of therapeutic interest. In this study, we evaluated the in vitro cytotoxic anti-tumor and immunomodulatory activities and in vivo anti-tumor effect of Laser Activated Calendula Extract (LACE), a novel extract of the plant

Calendula Officinalis. The results indicate that LACE aqueous extract has two complementary activities in vitro with potential anti-tumor therapeutic effect: cytotoxic tumor cell activity and lymphocyte activation. The suppressive effects of LACE extract produced a ranged from 70 to 100%.

Herbal Product Suppliers

Gaia Herbs
108 Island Ford Road,
Brevard, NC 28712
(828) 884-4242
www.gaiaherbs.com

Herbalists and Alchemist
PO Box 553
Broadway, NJ 08808
(908) 689-9092

Herb Pharm
PO Box 116
Williams, OR 97544
(800) 348-4372
www.herb-pharm.com

Mountain Rose Herbs
PO Box 50220
Eugene, OR 97405
(800) 879-3337
www.mountainroseherbs.com

Wise Woman Herbals
PO Box 270
Creswell, OR 97426
541.895.5172
www.wisewomanherbals.com

References

Anderson, RA. (2001). *Clinician's guide to holistic medicine.* Chicago: McGraw Hill.

Angele, MK, Schwacha, MG, Ayala, A, Chaudry, IH. (2000)Effect of gender and sex hormones on immune responses following shock. *Shock*, 14(2):81-90.

Aria, MH, Duarte, AJ, and Natale, VM. (2006). The effects of long-term endurance training on the immune and endocrine systems of elderly men: the role of cytokines and anabolic hormones. *Immune Ageing.* Aug 25;3:9.

Balch, Phyllis and James. (2000). *Prescriptions for Nutritional Healing,* (3rd ed.). New York: Avery.

Baltrusch HJ, Stangel W, Titze I. (1991). Stress, cancer and immunity. New developments in biopsychosocial and psychoneuroimmunologic research. Acta neurologica. Aug;13(4):315-27.

Belpoggi, F et al. (2006). First experimental demonstration of the multipotential carcinogenic effects of aspartame administered in the feed to Sprague-Dawley rats. *Environmental Health Perspectives.* 114, 379-85.

Berczi, I. (1997). Pituitary hormones and immune function. *Acta Paediatrica Suppl*, 423:70-5.

Body Ecology. *A tale of incredible sweetness and intrigue.* Retrieved May 15, 2007, from http://www.stevia.net/html

Boonkaewwan C, Toskulkao C, Vongsakul M. (2006). Anti-Inflammatory and Immunomodulatory Activities of Stevioside and Its Metabolite Steviol on THP-1 Cells. *Journal of Agriculture and Food Chemistry*, 8;54(3):785.

Bove, Mary. (2001). *An encyclopedia of natural healing for children and infants.* Chicago: Keats.

Bremzen, AV and Welchman, J. (1995). *Terrific Pacific Cookbook.* New York: Workman Publishing.

Cavanaugh, Christopher. (2001). Strengthen Your Immune System. *The Reader's Digest Association.*

Colic, M and Savic, M. (2000). Garlic extracts stimulate proliferation of rat lymphocytes in vitro by increasing IL-2 and IL-4 production. *Immunopharmacology and Immunotoxicology.* Feb;22(1):163-81.

Cooking Live. *Sweet Potato Soup.* Retrieved March 15, 2007 from http://www.foodnetwork.com/food/recipes/recipe/0,1977,FOOD _9936_13378,00.html

Dickstein JB, Moldofsky H. (1999). Sleep, cytokines and immune function. *Sleep Medicine Review,* 3(3):219-28.

Dorshkind, K and Horseman, ND. (2000). The roles of prolactin, growth hormone, insulin-like growth factor-I, and thyroid hormones in lymphocyte development and function: insights from genetic models of hormone and hormone receptor deficiency. *Endocrine Reviews.* 21(3): 292-312.

Dreher, H. (1995). *The immune power personality.* New York: Dutton.

Emsellem, HA and Whiteley, C. (2006). *Snooze or Lose: No war ways to improve your teen's sleep habits.* Washington, DC: Joseph Henry Press.

Environmental Protection Agency. *Plants That Promote Clean Air.* Retrieved May 15, 2007, from http://www.epa.gov/html

Food news report card. Retrieved 4/12/2006 from http://www.foodnews.org/reportcard.php

Garriga, MM and Metcalfe, DD. (1988) Aspartame intolerance. *Annals of Allergy.* Dec;61:63-9.

Gelfand, EW et al. (2003). The hygiene hypothesis revisited: Pros and cons. 60th Anniversary Meeting of the *American Academy of Allergy, Asthma and Immunology*

Gladstar, Rosemary. (1993). *Herbal healing for women.* New York: Fireside.

Grimsley, E, Patel, RM, Sarma, R. (2006). Popular sweetener Sucralose as a migraine trigger. *Annals of Allergy*,46(8):1303-4

Hartung, T. (2000).*Growing 101 Herbs That Heal: Gardening techniques, recipes and remedies.* Pownal, VT: Storey Book Publishing.

Himalayan International Institute of Yoga Science and Philosophy. (1994). *Neti Pot.* Honesdale, PA.

Holmes, TH and Rahe, RH. The social readjustment rating scale. *Journal of Psychosomatic Research*, 11:213-213.

Infante-Rivard C, Labuda D, Krajinovic M, Sinnett D. (1999). Risk of childhood leukemia associated with exposure to pesticides and with gene polymorphisms. *Epidemiology*, 10:481-7.

International College of Integrative Medicine. (2002) Chelation Therapy Workshop, March. Tampa Florida.

International Food Information Council. (2004). *Sugar alcohol fact sheet.* Retrieved June 15, 2007, from http://http://www.ific.org/publications/factsheets/sugaralcoholfs.cfm

Irwin, M et al. (1996). Partial night sleep deprivation reduces natural killer and cellular immune responses in humans. *The FASEB Journal.* Apr 10(5):643-53.

Janele, D. et al. (2006). Effects of testosterone, 17beta-estradiol, and downstream estrogens on cytokine secretion from human leukocytes in the presence and absence of cortisol. *Annals of the New York Academy of Sciences,* 1069:168-82

Jessop, et al (2001). Resistance to glucocorticoid feedback in obesity. *Journal of Clinical Endocrinology and Metabolism*. 86: 4109–4114.

Kalra R, Singh SP, Savage SM, Finch GL, Sopori ML. (2000). Effects of cigarette smoke on immune response: chronic exposure to cigarette smoke impairs antigen-mediated signaling in T cells and depletes IP3-sensitive $Ca(2+)$ stores. *Journal of Pharmacology and Experimental Therapeutics*.Apr;293(1):166-71.

Khorram, O. Vu, L, Yen, SS. (1997). Activation of immune function by dehydroepiandrosterone (DHEA) in age-advanced men. *Journal of Gerontology*, 52(1):M1-7.

Lair, C. (1997). *Feeding the whole family: Whole foods recipes for babies, young children and their parents.* Seattle: Moon Smile Press.

Lehey, Stephen. (2006) New studies back benefit of organic diet. *Interpress Services* retrieved May 11, 2006 from http://www.organicconsumers.org/2006/article_91.cfm

Lu C, et al. (2006). Organic diets significantly lower children's dietary exposure to organophosphorus pesticides. *Environmental Health Perspectives*. 114: 260-263.

Makinen, KK et al. (1995). Xylitol chewing gums and caries rates: a 40-month cohort study. *Journal of Dental Research*. 74: 1904-13.

Marz, RB. (1999). *Medical nutrition from marz* (2nd ed.). Portland: Omni-Press.

Murray, MT. (1993). *The healing power of foods*. Rocklin, CA: Prima Publishing.

National Center for Immunization and Respiratory Diseases/Division of Bacterial Diseases. (2006). *Get smart: Know when antibiotic work.* Retrieved January 23, 2007, from

http://www.cdc.gov/drugresistance/community/anitbiotic-
resistance.htm.

National Institute on Alcohol Abuse and Alcoholism.(1993)
Alcohol Alert. 22. PH 346.

Niemela, M, Kontiokari, T and Uhari, M. (1998). A novel use
of xylitol sugar in preventing acute otitis media. *Pediatrics.* 102:
879-84.

Nieman, DC. (1997). Exercise immunology: practical
applications. International Journal of Sports Medicine. Supp 1
1:S91-100.

Sanchez A, et al. (1973). Role of sugars in human
neutrophilic phagocytosis. *American Journal of Clinical
Nutrition,* 26(11):1180-4.

Shealy, NC. (1999). *DHEA, the youth and health hormone.*
Chicago: Keats.

Taste of History Cookbook. Friends of Hot Springs Public
Library Building Fund Raiser.

Tierra, L. (2000). *A kids herb book.* San Francisco, CA:
Robert. R. Reed Publishing.

U.S. Department of Agriculture, Agricultural Research
Service. (2005). *USDA National Nutrient Database for Standard
Reference,* Release 18. Retrieved February 20, 2007, from
http://www.nal.usda.gov/fnic/foodcomp.

Wang, HC, and Klein, JR. (2001).Immune function of thyroid
stimulating hormone and receptor. *Critical Review of
Immunology,* 21(4): 323-37.

Watzl, B. et al. (2004). Daily moderate amounts of red wine
or alcohol have no effect on the immune system of healthy men
European Journal of Clinical Nutrition. Jan;58(1):40-5.

Wiegert DA, Blalock JE. (1987). Interactions between the neuroendocrine and immune systems: common hormones and receptors. *Immunological Review*, 100:79-108.

Winston, D. (2006). *Herbal approaches to autoimmune disease*. Proceeding of the 17th Annual AHG Symposium: Boulder, CO.

Young, Kay. (1993). *Wild Seasons: Gathering and Cooling Wild Plants of the Great Plains*. Lincoln, NE: University of Nebraska Press.

Youngblood, C. (1999). *Advanced Topics in Herbal Medicine Notes*. Seattle: Bastyr University.

Zahn SH, Ward MH.(1998). Pesticides and childhood cancer. *Environmental Health Perspectives*, 106 Suppl **3**:893-908.

Index

About the Author

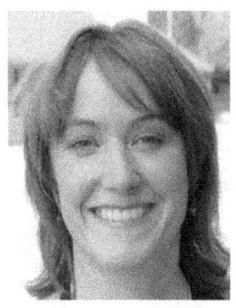 **Faith A. Christensen, ND** is a Naturopathic Physician in private practice in the Colorado Springs area specializing in Women's and Children's Health. Dr. Christensen earned a four year doctorate in Naturopathic Medicine from Bastyr University, the "Harvard" of naturopathic medical schools, a BA in Botany from the University of Washington and an Associate in Nursing from Excelsior College.

Dr. Christensen founded and operated a successful naturopathic clinic in Seattle for several years, and also practiced in Chicago before moving to Colorado Springs. Dr. Christensen focuses on the structural, nutritional, mental, and emotional aspects of health.

She strives to find the cause of illness through careful history taking, functional blood work, salivary hormone testing, digestive stool analysis, food allergy testing, and neuro-transmitter testing. She encourages each patient to find wholeness in all aspects of life, and empowers people to take charge of their health.

She has taught craniosacral therapy since 1998 through Integrated Bodywork Institute, VIS Medicine, and as an adjunct faculty at Bastyr University. She has published five manuals for various craniosacral classes and lectures across the country on health and bodywork. To contact Dr. Christensen, visit www.vitavisweb.com.